Responding to the Challenge

Responding to the Challenge

Current Trends and International Issues in Developmental Disabilities

Essays in Honor of Gunnar Dybwad

Hank Bersani Jr., Ph.D.
Editor

Brookline Books

Copyright ©1999 by Brookline Books, Inc.

All rights reserved. No part of this work covered by the copyright hereon may be reproduced or used in any form or by any means — graphic, electronic, or mechanical, including photocopying, recording, taping, or information storage and retrieval systems — without the permission of the publisher.

Library of Congress Cataloging-in-Publication Data
Responding to the challenge : current issues and international
　developments in developmental disabilities : essays in honor of
　Gunnar Dybwad / Hank Bersani, Jr., editor.
　　p.　cm.
　Includes bibliographical references and index.
　ISBN 1-57129-075-3
　1. Mentally handicapped.　2. Developmentally disabled.
I. Dybwad, Gunnar.　II. Bersani, Hank A.
HV3004.R455　1999
362.1;968–dc21　　　　　　　　　　　　　　　99-35778
　　　　　　　　　　　　　　　　　　　　　　　　CIP

Cover design by Kate Rubin.
Printed in USA by R.R. Donnelley & Sons.

Published by
BROOKLINE BOOKS
P.O. Box 1047
Cambridge, MA 02238-1047
(617) 868-0360
Within the USA, order toll-free: 1-800-666-BOOK

Contents

Acknowledgments .... *ix*
Foreword .... *xi*
Stanley S. Herr
In Celebration of Gunnar Dybwad .... *xiii*
Hank Bersani, Jr.
Editor's Preface .... *xvii*

SECTION I: CONCEPTUAL ISSUES

1 **The Medical Model** 3
   A Mostly Historical Discussion
   Allen C. Crocker

2 **The Role of Science in Advancing the Lives of People with Intellectual Disabilities** 10
   Trevor R. Parmenter, Ph.D.

3 **Architectural Trends and Values** 23
   From Humanizing Institutions to Inclusive Communities
   Elaine Ostroff

4 **The Metaphor of Mental Retardation** 35
   Rethinking Ability and Disability
   Douglas Biklen

SECTION II: LEGAL ISSUES

5 **From Deficiency to Equality** 55
   How are Canada's New Constitutional Protections Working for Persons with Disabilities?
   Orville Endicott

6 **The Rights Revolution** 69
   From Isolation To Wyatt, Wyoming, And Beyond
   Stanley S. Herr

7 **On the Closing of Mansfield Training School** 91
   Robert Perske

SECTION III: INTERNATIONAL ISSUES

8 **People with Mental Retardation and Europe 2000** 97
   Comparing Cultural Trends and Different Experiences
   Ann-Margrethe Brandt

9 **Getting There** 104
   How Are We Doing Internationally?
   Walter Eigner & Helmut Spudich

10 **Overcoming Challenges of Organizational Retardation** 109
   A Convoluted Approach to Addressing the Eye Care Needs of People with Mental Retardation in Israel
   Richard E. Isralowitz, Ph.D.

11 Meeting the Challenge of Intellectual Disability 116
    An International Perspective
    Peter Mittler

12 Discussion on the Future Design of Residential Care for Persons with
    Mental Retardation in Japan 123
    Akihiko Takahashi, M.D.

13 The 'Lebenshilfe' in Germany 127
    Tom Mutters

14 The Situation of Mentally Handicapped Persons and Their Families in
    Eastern Europe 133
    Tom Mutters

SECTION IV: SELF-ADVOCACY ISSUES

15 On Being Left Out 145
    Barb Goode

16 Gentle Words To Self-Advocate Friends 147
    Robert Perske

17 Who Teaches Us? 151
    Michael J. Kennedy

18 Tokenism—It Doesn't Look Good!!! 155
    Liz Obermayer

19 Who Speaks for Whom? 158
    Issues of Advocacy
    Ann Shearer & Alison Wertheimer

20 Not to Yield 164
    Robert Williams Parsons Cutler, Jr.

SECTION V: FAMILY ISSUES

21 An Unanticipated Life: 173
    The Impact of Lifelong Caregiving
    Marty Wyngaarden Krauss & Marsha Mailick Seltzer

22 Gender, Disability, and Community Life 189
    Toward a Feminist Analysis
    Rannveig Traustadóttir

23 In Her Own Home 207
    The Experiences of Catherine Schaefer
    Zana Marie Lutfiyya

SECTION VI: CONCLUSION

24 Impatience, Mountains and the Moon 215
    Gerald Provencal

    Appendix 1: Curriculum Vitae of Gunnar Dybwad 229
    Appendix 2: Concluding Remarks from Gunnar Dybwad 231
    Appendix 3: A Final Tribute to Rosemary F. Dybwad, Ph.D. 233
    About the Editor 239

With thanks to Sr. Janice Ryan, who recruited me,
and in memory of Burton Blatt who trained me,
and in loving memory of Rosemary F. Dybwad — you are missed.

Acknowledgments

A volume of over 300 pages, with 25 chapters from 10 countries and several continents does not just happen.

The production of this volume was an honor and a pleasure, which would not have been possible without the efforts, and graciousness of so many people.

To the authors, many of whom I have never met, thank you for your eagerness, and your diligence.

To the publisher, thanks for your patience when it was needed, and for your gentle prodding when that was needed.

To my colleagues at work, thank you as well. Melanie and Tina for your understanding, and Maxine for your practical assistance.

Finally, my deepest gratitude to my family, Lynda, Lisa and Alex who were always understanding when I had to back out on a family outing because I was working on what our household has come to call "Gunnar's book."

— H.B.

Foreword

Stanley S. Herr

As the millennium approaches, the drive to define and implement legal and human rights remains a hallmark of the disabilities field. Gunnar Dybwad has proven to be one of the larger figures in that campaign. Ten years ago in a speech on his 80th birthday, I sketched his influence in these terms:

Gunnar's description of his career as a "long and fruitful collaboration" with attorneys is only one element of his being a godfather to people involved with the disabilities field.

As both a doer and a thinker, he made sense out of complexity and provided hope that we could undo the horror of human abuse. He dared us to believe the formerly unthinkable: the end of institutions and the rise of self-advocacy.

In 1971, when I first contacted Gunnar to provide an affidavit in *Mills v. Board of Education* [which would become a landmark case on ensuring the right to free, appropriate education], he was the only expert who could write a statement that was memorable, crisp, and bold. He compared giving children two hours of instruction per week to giving a starving child two meals a week. Just as two meals a week do not make a diet, he explained, so two hours of instruction do not make an educational program for a child with a disability.

In *Wyatt v. Stickney* in 1972, Gunnar used his own initiative in bringing to Judge Johnson's attention the U.N. Declaration of the Rights of Mentally Retarded Persons [1971]. Thankfully, Gunnar did not first ask me or the other lawyers for our opinion or advice. We would have never predicted that the judge would use the U.N. Declaration to support a right to habilitation.

In 1973, Gunnar stood with Mr. Arrol Townsend and his plaintiff cohorts, who had endured a form of servitude in Tennessee's institutions, and urged justice and compensation for them. [See *Townsend v. Clover Bottom Hospital and School*, 1978] He did all of this while some of his fellow experts were shamefully refusing to testify because of political pressure or new found ambivalence.

I could continue in a similar vein year by year. But the point is clear. A list of Gunnar's accomplishments and contributions in legal arenas could continue for pages. The point however, is that Gunnar Dybwad has always been there when an oppressed person was in need. Gunnar and his wife Rosemary were never too busy to offer a word of encouragement, comment on a manuscript, or provide hospitality to a wandering scholar. Truly he became a force for good in my life and in the lives of so many others![1]

Although Professor Dybwad might resist this or other accolades, the historical record and the privileges of authorship fully justify this introduction. The man and the movement for equal rights for people with disabilities are clearly intertwined.

In Celebration of Gunnar Dybwad

In the fall of 1976, I enrolled in a course titled "International Issues in Special Education and Rehabilitation" at Syracuse University. The professor, a gentle man, had an interpersonal style and warmth that belied our stereotype based on his Germanic accent. His energy, zest for life, and love of hard work and long days belied his age — quite old to many of us. He was after all a man of 67 years who flew once a week from Boston before dawn to spend the day teaching, mentoring, and supporting students in a university hundreds of miles from his home.

The Special Education Department, headed by Burton Blatt, was already famous for its luminaries, but I heard these other professors extol the virtues of Professor Dybwad. "National leader," they said. "Influenced much of the history of the last 30 years," we were told. "Still has a clear vision and sense of direction to offer the field." This old professor. A quiet, modest man with a bow-tie, a goatee, and his hair parted solidly in the middle of his head.

It has been my pleasure to work with Dr. Dybwad Professor Emeritus of Human Development at the Heller School of Brandeis University, since the formative years of my career. Those of us that have had the pleasure to experience his impact "up close and personal" call him "The Old Professor."

Dr. Dybwad, now in his 90th year, remembers from personal experience the major accomplishments of the past 65 years. In fact, he was a major player in building the organizations, passing the legislation and deciding the litigation that shaped the development of rehabilitation and human services as we know them today.

Dr. Dybwad's impact on the literature of our field began early. By 1964, as the director of the organization then known as the National Association for Retarded Children, Dr. Dybwad had published numerous major papers and given countless important addresses that the Columbia University Press published as a collection of his most influential papers. *The Challenge of Mental Retardation* included essays such as "Are we retarding the retarded?" Originally published in 1960, this essay was an indictment of low quality services which forced low expectancies and stereotypes on people with cognitive impairments. As a doctoral student in 1976, I remember how I marveled at how current of the volume still seemed, 16 years later.

In 1969, Dybwad published *Action Implication: The USA Today.* In that paper he called for better training and pay for direct care staff, cited the important role of citizen volunteers, stressed the value of employment, and called for the closure of residential institutions. Nearly 30 years old, it is still a manifesto for activists today.

More recently, I had the opportunity to assist The Old Professor in editing *New Voices: Self-Advocacy by People with Disabilities.* In this book, he presents some 21 chapters about the emergence of self-advocacy across the globe. Chapters are written by authors from Australia and Austria, Sweden and England, Canada and the US.

Considered by many to be the great-grandfather of the self-advocacy movement, Gunnar Dybwad has had a greater influence on the lives of people with disabilities than probably anyone else alive today. In 1995, writing in praise of self-advocates as teachers, he wrote: "So how can we understand and help these people who call themselves self-advocates? Only by watching them — simply watching them and cheering them on."

The Old Professor's travel schedule would tire a person of half his years as he responds to his many constituencies across the globe. In three months at the age of 87, he made two trips to Europe to speak. In July, his trip focused on England, but one day he was scheduled to speak in Paris to UNESCO. Not a problem for The Old Professor. In the morning, he took a train through the new "Chunnel" (the tunnel under the English Channel), gave his speech in Paris, and returned for an evening in London with his hosts.

On the second trip, in September, he flew to Prague to speak at the first international human rights conference to be held in the new Czech Republic. Later that week he gave an address to the national People First group in Austria. By the end of the week, he was in Geneva speaking at a human rights conference sponsored by the International League of Societies for Persons with Intellectual Handicaps, which was co-sponsored by the United Nations Human Rights Organization. In between, he was a guest speaker at a conference sponsored by the Presidents Committee on Mental Retardation.

We literally do not have the space here to recount all of the awards and recognition that Dr. Dybwad has received on his own and in collaboration with his wife, Rosemary. The walls of the family home, including the basement, are lined with proclamations signed by presidents and international figures, photographs with President Kennedy and other governmental leaders.

He is a Fellow in the American Association on Mental Retardation, the American Sociological Association, the American Orthopsychiatric Association, and the American Public Health Association. He is also an honorary Fellow of the American Academy of Pediatrics. Most recently, the national Association on Mental Retardation renamed their humanitarian award the "Gunnar Dybwad Humanitarian Award."

During their career together, Rosemary and Gunnar Dybwad traveled the globe consulting in more than 30 nations. Together they were goodwill ambassadors known in disability rights circles throughout the world. While Gunnar was Executive Director of the National Arc, Rosemary assisted in the formation of the International League of Societies for Persons with Mental Handicaps, a worldwide organization of parents that continues to be an inter-national force today, working closely with the United Nations to support the rights and inclusion of people with cognitive disabilities throughout the world.

A number of years ago, at the suggestion of Gunnar and Rosemary, I was touring services in Norway and Sweden. As I found my way around both countries, many professionals and government leaders with busy schedules agreed to meet with me and be interviewed by yet another American visitor. Whenever things were not going well, I would find a way to work in the conversation that my study tour was formulated at the urging of Gunnar and Rosemary. Without exception, from parents of adults with disabilities to top bureaucrats, the response was "You know the Dybwads?", usually followed by "Can you come to our home for dinner?" I lost track of the amount of hospitality that was extended to me over my three weeks of travel whenever I mentioned Gunnar and Rosemary. The next year, I visited Australia, and once again mention of the magic name "Dybwad" opened doors for me as a traveling stranger.

A few years ago, Rosemary died, and The Old Professor continues to live in the house that was their home for so many years. He continues to tend the garden, not because he is a gardener, but because it is "Rosemary's Garden."

He continues to share his vision, generosity and humanity to all who cross his path.

Thank you *Old Professor* — a great leader, a renowned visionary and a good friend.

— Hank Bersani, Jr.

Editor's Preface

Hank Bersani, Jr.

In order for the reader to fully appreciate the power of this volume, a few notes are in order.

The title. In 1964, professor Dybwad published a powerful volume: *Challenges in Mental Retardation.* In 1997, when we began planning this book, I re-read as much of Dybwad's work as I could find. While it was all striking, the words from 1964 rang clear and true as if they were written today. Even the language is remarkably acceptable by our current ever-so-careful standards. I thought, if we are to celebrate the life of Dr. Dybwad, that a fitting format would be to explore how well our accomplishments of the last 30 years match up with the challenges that Dybwad so carefully posed to us in that volume.

A festschrift. A *festschrift* is a volume in celebration of an individual or an event of great importance or influence. This volume is a festschrift in honor of the life-work of Professor Dybwad, and in special recognition of his 90th birthday, July 12, 1999. It is not a book about him; there is little biography to be found in these pages. Rather, it is a reflection of ripples moving across the water. Dybwad made a splash in 1964, and the ripples were the push behind the careers of each of us in this volume.

The authors. There was no shortage of authors hoping, wishing, demanding to be contributors to this volume. And there was tremendous energy to create a book of praises for the man, and to shine a spotlight on the specifics of his career. However, the purpose of this volume is to give praise by indirect light. The authors were selected because they are active in areas inspired by Professor Dybwad and his wife, Rosemary, pursuing challenges laid out in 1964 which are still relevant today. The work they describe has been inspired by his teaching, and most often by his direct personal mentoring. In the measurement terminology so in vogue today, we are his outcome measures.

The cover. The artwork on the cover, is a Martha Perske drawing depicting Professor Dybwad on a visit to the infamous Willowbrook State Institution in New York. Although Perske is famous for her positive, uplifting drawings of people with disabilities in dignified poses, this one work stands out. Stark and to the point, she captures the sadness that was Willowbrook — and all institutions, and equally, the gracious dignity which Professor Dybwad shows everyone he meets regardless of their label or social standing.

The content. The content of the book is gathered into several topical areas. Each chapter stands alone. Together with the others in their section, they paint a broader picture, and all told, they present a mural — the big picture. This is not a volume that needs to be read sequentially. The reader can easily select a section to begin with, or an individual author, or a specific title. The topics may seem eclectic, but they all bear the same characteristic — they were inspired by the same man and his wife!

About writing styles. This volume is not the work of a single pen, and no efforts have been made to achieve stylistic homogeneity. Professor Dybwad has always valued diversity in his thinking, in his colleagues, and so in this volume. Many professions and disciplines are represented here, because Dr. Dybwad was active in so many professions and disciplines. The lawyers write like lawyers; the educators, more like educators, and the advocates like true advocates. Many of the authors are writing in their second (or third) language. Some are "professional" writers, some are self-advocates with little or no authoring experience. Editing has been limited to the most basic form. Spelling has been corrected, but international differences have been respected ("UK" spelling in chapters from the UK, Australia, and Canada). Labels, for the most part have been left as the authors wrote them. Thus, some refer to *intellectual disability,* while others refer to people with *mental retardation.* We trust that the reader will appreciate the individual flavors of the writing.

Two of the chapters include writing done by facilitated communication. In Biklen's chapter, quotes from people using facilitated communication are included in a different typeface. They have been edited for typographical errors as any other author, but we exerted great care not to edit. the tone to content of their writing. Cutler wrote his chapter using facilitated communication and it is presented in a different font as well as the work of the other self advocates who wrote in their own voice. Their work was also edited for the obvious typos, but no more.

SECTION I

Conceptual Issues

1

The Medical Model
A Mostly Historical Discussion

Allen C. Crocker
Harvard Medical School, Boston, MA

Personal Opening Note

The present discourse is given in gratitude to Gunnar Dybwad, who received me many years ago as a brash young medical colleague and who then patiently guided me into reasonable behaviors. In earlier times I could not have perceived the varied feelings and lore that surrounded the history of medical involvement in the field of mental retardation. I had no real idea that the term "medical model" had largely perjorative overtones (in certain usage situations). With Gunnar's help I have gradually come to appreciate the complexity of work in human exceptionality and the tentativeness with which all of the professions provide their contributions. Seen in an extended perspective medical input has often, of course, had seminal value, and in other settings has had an undistinguished role. In this tract I shall explore some past and current implications of the expression, medical model, as used in developmental disabilities, and attempt to underline the values in our common striving.

SOME THOUGHTS ABOUT THE MEDICAL PROCESS

Medical workers had a long way to come, to travel from the negative gradient of the early pediatric texts. One found comments like "The symptoms usually met with ... are the vacant expression, the occasional presence of strabismus, the drooping head,

---

Preparation of this material was supported in part by the US Department of Health and Human Services, Maternal and Child Health Bureau (Project MCJ-259150), and Administration on Developmental Disabilities (Project 90DD0357).

Acknowledgement is also expressed for assistance to Ms. Alison Clapp, Librarian at Children's Hospital, Boston; Mss. Bonnie Stecher and Robin Booth, Librarians at the Samuel Gridley Howe Library, Walter E. Fernald State School; and Mss. Margaret Chow-Menzer (General Counsel) and Gail Grossman (Quality Assurance), Massachusetts Department of Mental Retardation.

the drooling, and the lack of all idea of cleanliness" (Rotch, 1901). Adult texts did not even deal at all in these areas. As Gunnar pointed out 7 decades later, the academic pediatric establishment had remained derelict in their educational resolve for young trainees: "Many medical authorities still feel that the best places for the future practicing physician to hear about the management of patients with mental retardation are the large state institutions" (Dybwad, 1974). Further, until the time of the last two decades a possibly well-meaning but assuredly nonsearching philosophy among some pediatricians supported sustained admission of certain young children with developmental disabilities to state residential institutions, a practice that Gunnar decried (1974). And it remained for the "right to treatment" provisions of Section 504 of the Vocational Rehabilitation Act, Public Law 93-112 (regulations available in 1977) to assure full supports for survival for some newborn infants with multiple congenital anomalies (cf Baby Doe in Indiana in 1982).

Many parents, and other nonclinical colleagues, may have found poor identification of physicians on occasion with the real circumstances and needs of persons with mental retardation. Attitudes were sometimes thought to be patronizing, and diagnostic terminology was not kind. Until recent years many physicians had relatively little experience carrying out problem-solving in the setting of an interdisciplinary team, and this, too, complicated the effort for centers to achieve holistic planning for clients with retardation (Crocker, 1998). All of these factors, which are elements in the gradual evolution and improvement of medical education, have probably added somewhat to public uncertainty about the "medical model."

STATE RESIDENTIAL FACILITIES

Perhaps the most tangible representation of the "medical model" in mental retardation had been the assumption by physicians of administrative leadership of the state institutions (residential facilities). The circumstances of persons with mental retardation were addressed by early psychiatrists and neurologists (such as Esquirol and Seguin), with the development of special schools. A Boston physician, Samuel Gridley Howe, began in 1848, as a training center, what was to become Fernald State School, the first such facility in the U.S. This movement grew, with directorship commonly taken by physicians (usually psychiatrists). As Gunnar said, "psychiatrists claimed monopolistic control of mental retardation institutions" (Dybwad, 1964). What is now the principal multidisciplinary organization in the U.S. for professionals working in mental retardation was begun in 1876 as the Association of Medical Officers of American Institutions for Idiotic and Feebleminded Persons. In its first 30 years almost all of its presidents were M.D.'s (including Seguin and Fernald). The name was changed in 1906 to the American Association for the Study of the Feebleminded; this largely superintendents' organization was then led by physicians for most of the next 27 years. Later, as it became the American Association on Mental Deficiency (1933) it was less for superintendents and less medical (35% of its presidents were physicians) and yet later (1987) it was the American Association on Mental Retardation, with no further physician presidents.

In Massachusetts it had been required since the 19th century that the state school superintendents be physicians. This was continued, with the provision added in the 1960s that there be board certification in psychiatry, neurology, internal medicine, or pediatrics. In 1971 an earned doctorate was still required, but this could be in any discipline appropriate to the care, treatment, and education of persons with mental retardation. By 1986, the superintendents merely needed for qualification such educational and administrative experience as was determined by the commissioner to be necessary for the performance of duties.

As the early decades proceeded of physician leadership for state residential facilities there was concurrently a compliance of institutional design to the "medical model." This was described by Wolfensberger (1972), who noted that hierarchies of physicians and nurses were in charge, living areas were called nursing units or wards, residents were referred to as patients, resident care was called nursing care, and records were charts. In those days, hospital-type routines often prevailed, nursing stations had large central spaces, various other caretaker personnel might have uniforms, and many nonmedical policy decisions were made by physicians. By 1975, Scheerenberger reported that fewer states were requiring a medical degree for the superintendent. He diagrammed as well the "Traditional Nonmedical Model" and the "Standard Unit Approach" for state residential facilities. That it was useful to designate a "Nonmedical Model" demonstrates the degree of residual medical influence. In recent times it has been usual to title the doctor who is the clinical chief as "Director of Medical Services" rather than the former term, "Medical Director," to reduce confusing roles.

Massachusetts had a unified state agency for many years, with a Commissioner of Mental Health and an Assistant Commissioner for Mental Retardation. Both were required by statute to be physicians. An acceptable credential for the Assistant Commissioner was added in 1966 to include being a diplomat from the American Board of Examiners in Professional Psychology. In 1986, Mental Retardation became a full department. It was then required only that the new commissioner "possess such educational qualifications and such administrative and other experience (including education or experience in a field related to human services) as the secretary of human services determines is necessary for performance of the duties for commissioner" (G.L. c. 19B).

THE MEDICAL MODEL AS IT HAS RELATED TO DISABILITY

The traditional core of concern regarding medical roles or views in the area of developmental disabilities involves what is called "medicalization" or the "medical model of disability." These two associated phenomena had complex historic dynamics, many benign, but came to symbolize a physician or medical service assumptiveness that was disturbing.

Bradley (1994) identifies the late 1960s as the era when medical leadership in service design began to modulate (when what was being called the medical model began to evolve into the developmental model). In the period before this there was commonly a biomedical conceptualization of the dilemma of the person with a disability that served to restrict the image of that person. Wolfensberger (1972) catches this most tellingly when he speaks of there having been the perception of "the deviant individual as sick".*

The most critical objection with over-emphasizing the possible organic origins of a disability is the tendency thereby to portray the predominant problem as located within the individual, who emerges then as abnormal or inferior — "that there are things *wrong* with people with disabilities" (Bickenbach, 1992). Expressed another way, although it is obvious that the difficulties confronting a person who is blind are substantially the product of a non-accommodating social environment, in the medical model there would be an inclination to believe that the "real problem" is not social but is an abnormality of the blind person himself (Bickenbach, 1992).

There is a danger that medical labeling of persons with disabilities will center on prognostic implications, and fail to regard the individual flexibly in holistic and functional considerations. Fitzgerald (1997) calls this biologic determinism, and notes that it is one way of "other-ing" people. A biomedical origin may raise elements of "the personal tragedy theory," and query about possible obligation to seek a curative intervention (Imrie, 1997).

Beyond the destiny and tragedy overtones there is also the issue of the sphere of control in medicalization of disability. Zola has pointed out eloquently that medical claims of special knowledge and judgment have often tended toward excessive management behaviors (1977). He states that medical workers may attach a label or insinuation of illness to the circumstances of impairment in a rather immodest fashion. This process can occur "through the expansion of what in life is deemed relevant to the good practice of medicine, through retention of absolute control over certain technical procedures, ... and through the expansion of what in medicine is deemed relevant to the good practice of life." Areas for conjecture relating to persons with disabilities also include such constituents as psychotropic medications, reproductive rights, reconstructive surgery, and end-of-life care.

Writing back at the time of much transition, Philip Roos (1971) offered a thoughtful commentary on "misinterpreting criticisms of the Medical Model" (and he always capitalized the words). In his view the troubling components included (1) defining mental retardation as an illness, (2) structuring the relationship between professionals and clients in terms of healer-patient roles, and (3) stressing the impor-

---

* He also notes some terms of other origin that were also used on occasion, including the deviant individual as "an object of pity," "an eternal child," or "a burden of charity."

tance of diagnosis and prognosis. He rushed to point out that criticism of the Medical Model, on the other hand, in no way implies opposition to "good medical care" (!) And he also defended some medical administrators as not necessarily specifically involved with Medical Model considerations.

It is of interest that the well-known nosologic system, the "ICIHD" (International Classification of Impairments, Disabilities, and Handicaps), organized as a supplement to the WHO International Classification of Diseases, is considered by some as a part of the "medicalization of disablement" because of its orientation by disease (Marks, 1997). The provisions of the Americans with Disabilities Act, on the other hand, are built on the understanding that a disabling condition is particularly a state of society itself, not a physical or mental state (Silvers, 1996).

Zola (1991) noted that there can be a utility in a medical identification with disability in that medical budgets for items like social support and assistive devices may prove relatively more stable when cuts are threatened in benefit provisions. Krauss (1993) urges caution in this regard. "To what extent," she asks, "is the need to transform life necessities into 'health care' simply an expedient option to obtain fiscal assistance for what could more legitimately be categorized as family support?" Health dollars transform typical *daily needs* for persons with atypical characteristics (such as mental retardation) into *events* supervised by medical personnel and regulated by bureaucrats, she surmises. Achieving balance can be difficult. Some persons with disabilities may find help in their home feasible when a managed care policy gives coverage, but lost when there is changeover to Medicaid, which may not be able, for example, to support in-home medication administration (Johnson, 1999).

INDEPENDENT LIVING

A significant piece of the medical model story relates to the Independent Living movement (IL). The IL crusade started in the late 1960s and early 1970s, largely by energetic and visionary students with disabilities separately in Champaign-Urbana, Berkeley, and Boston. They were determined to build consumer sovereignty, self-reliance, and political and economic rights. The ideas stand in contrast to discrimination and dependency. Likewise, they stand in contrast to the medical model, which views people as needing to be "cured" (NCOD, 1996).

It was implicit that the traditional medical configuration was unacceptable:

> The IL movement is very much a partisan in the medicalization/self-care debate. At issue is the extent to which the management of disability should remain under the aegis of the medical care system, once medical stability has been substantially obtained. Most public policies regarding disability require some type of professional medical presence, whether in the acute stages of disability, in the determination of benefits, or in long-term institutional care. The IL movement asserts that much of this medical presence is both unnecessary and counter-

productive. Central to the IL movement is the belief that the management of stabilized disabilities is primarily a personal matter and only secondarily a medical matter (DeJong, 1983).

Further, personal assistance (such as from PCAs), in the eyes of this disability rights movement, is an item of social liberation—just like a light-weight wheelchair or a bus lift—not a form of medical care (Shapiro, 1993).

Contact with Centers for Independent Living has served to teach many physicians about the deeper personal meaning of impairment, and about the need for building trust and shared effort. The IL movement has involved predominantly people with physical disabilities, providing counseling, education, and practical supports, but there is some application as well to individuals with sensory, mental health, or cognitive disability. Obviously many of the personal rights issues relate to persons well beyond the actual IL movement itself. It is in the area of health maintenance and prevention of secondary conditions that useful new dialogue and planning has begun.

WHERE ARE WE GOING?

The relationships described in this tract between medical workers and the disability world reveal an evolving alliance, with much learning. A lot of the misunderstanding is behind us. It is interesting to note that the characteristics of available health care for persons with disabilities is currently being extensively reviewed and reinforced, as management of medical contracts becomes a national preoccupation (Crocker, 1999). Consumer voices are also increasingly effective, and various types of practice guidelines from professional groups (including by textbooks) add to the capacity for quality improvement.

The knowledge base regarding diagnostic studies and intelligent clinical supports is in a greatly enhanced state. The fields of developmental and developmental-behavioral pediatrics are now each seeking the establishment of subspecialty board certification, and family medicine is assuming more responsibility in longterm care for persons with disability. Nurse practitioner contributions are pivotal in all sections of the country.

I would believe that the designation of medical model (and even of Medical Model!) is closer now to implying interactions that are accurate, with shared contributions and teamwork. Our grounding in human rights is germane (Crocker and Cushna, 1976) and the guiding ethical precepts are sturdy (Crocker, 1998).

References

Bickenbach JE. The biomedical model of disablement. In: Bickenbach JE, *Physical Disability and Social Policy*. Toronto: University of Toronto Press, 1992, pp 61-92

Bradley VJ. Evolution of a new service paradigm. In: Bradley VJ, Ashbaugh JW, Blaney BC, eds., *Creating Individual Supports for People with Developmental Disabilities*. Baltimore, Paul H. Brookes Publishing Co, 1994, pp 11-32

Crocker AC. Medicine. in: Orelove FP, Garner HG, eds., *Teamwork: Parents and Professionals Speak for Themselves*. Washington: CWLA Press, 1998, pp 55-71

Crocker AC. Community-based and managed health care. In: Wehmeyer M, Patton JR, eds. *Mental Retardation in the 21st Century*. Austin: PRO-ED, Inc., 1999

Crocker AC, Cushna B. Ethical considerations and attitudes in the field of developmental disorders. In: Johnston RB, Magrab PR, eds., *Developmental Disorders: Evaluation, Treatment, and Education*. Baltimore: University Park Press, 1976, pp 495-502

DeJong G. Defining and implementing the independent living concept. In: Crewe NM, Zola IK, and Associates, eds., *Independent Living for Physically Disabled People*. San Francisco: Jossey-Bass Publishers, 1983, pp 5-27

Dybwad G. *Challenges in Mental Retardation*. New York: Columbia University Press, 1964, p. 124

Dybwad G. Remarks on receiving the C. Anderson Aldrich Award. *Pediatrics*, 54:489, 1974

Fitzgerald F. Reclaiming the whole: Self, spirit, and society. *Disability and Rehabilitation*, 19:407, 1997

Imrie R. Rethinking the relationships between disability, rehabilitation, and society. *Disability and Rehabilitation*, 19:263, 1997

Johnson M. In thrall to the medical model. *Ragged Edge*, 20:12, 1999

Krauss MW. On the medicalization of family caregiving. Mental Retardation, 31:78, 1993

Marks D. Models of disability. *Disability and Rehabilitation*, 19:85, 1997

National Council on Disability. Independent living, disability rights, and disability culture. In: NCOD, *Achieving Independence: the Challenge for the 21st Century*. Washington: National Council on Disability, 1996, pp 17-22

Roos P. Misinterpreting criticisms of the medical model. *Mental Retardation*, 9:22, 1971

Rotch TM. *Pediatrics: The Hygienic and Medical Treatment of Children*, Third Edition, Philadelphia: J.B. Lippincott Co., 1901, p. 930

Scheerenberger RC. *Managing Residential Facilities for the Developmentally Disabled*. Springfield IL: Charles C. Thomas, Publisher, 1975, p. 116

Silvers A. (In)equality, (ab)normality, and the Americans with Disabilities Act. J. *Medicine & Philosophy*, 21:209, 1996

Wolfensberger W. *The Principle of Normalization in Human Services*. Toronto: National Institute on Mental Retardation, 1972, p. 68

Zola IK. Healthism and disabling medicalization. In: Illich I, Zola IK, McKnight J, Caplan J, Shaiken H (eds.), *Disabling Professions*. London: Marion Boyars, 1977, pp 41-67

Zola IK. The medicalization of aging and disability. *Advances in Medical Sociology*, 2:299, 1991

2

The Role of Science in Advancing the Lives of People with Intellectual Disabilities

Trevor R. Parmenter, Ph.D.
President, International Association for the Scientific Study of Intellectual Disabilities

This chapter will provide reflections upon the state of the art of research into intellectual disabilities[*] from an international perspective over the past 25 years. It will draw essentially from the activities of the International Association for the Scientific Study of Intellectual Disabilities (IASSID), whose Articles of Incorporation state that the general purpose of the Association, "is the world-wide promotion of the scientific study of intellectual and related developmental disabilities and of the conditions of persons with such disabilities and their families." Observations on future directions in research and the role IASSID might play will be made.

In terms of the history of the provision of services and inquiry into the needs, especially the educational needs, of people with disabilities, one must turn to Europe and the Nordic countries. Indeed, the recorded history of the care of people with disabilities goes back to the Middle Ages. For instance, a public hospital for blind people was established in France in 1260. In 1749, Pereire demonstrated before the Academy of Science in Paris his success in teaching congenitally deaf people to speak and read (July, 1981). The social and philosophical teachings of the Swiss-French reformer Jean-Jacques Rousseau which provided an impetus for the education of handicapped persons, it is suggested, also inspired Itard to commence his

---

[*] The term *intellectual disabilities* is becoming the more preferred term internationally as a synonym for mental retardation (USA), learning disabilities (U.K. and Ireland), mental handicap and mental deficiency. It is recognized that all labels have pejorative connotations and may be hurtful to people thus described.

The assistance of Noel Atkinson in the preparation of this chapter is gratefully acknowledged.
Author's address for correspondence: Centre for Developmental Disability Studies, PO Box 6, Ryde, NSW 1680, Australia.

famous attempt to teach the 'wild boy' of Aveyron. Itard's work subsequently influenced his pupil, Seguin, to develop educational materials for persons with intellectual disabilities. Other significant European figures who impacted on educational philosophies and methods include Pestalozzi, Guggenbühl, Braille, Froebel, Binet, Montessori, and Inhelder.

Notable immigrants from Europe who have influenced the USA scene include Bettelheim, Dreikurs, Redl, Dybwad, Frostig, Lovaas, Strauss and Wolfensberger; all of whom have made a significant impact upon service provisions for people with disabilities. In the United Kingdom, significant contributors to our field have included Tredgold, Burt, Tizard, Gunzberg, Kusshlick, Rutter and Clarke and Clarke. From the Nordic area, figures such as Bank-Mikkelsen, Nirje, Grunewald and Magne have had a profound influence on services internationally.

It was Edouard Seguin, who together with five colleagues, founded the American Association on Mental Deficiency (AAMD) in 1876, the centenary of the American Declaration of Independence. A century later, the Fourth Congress of the International Association for the Scientific Study of Mental Deficiency (IASSMD later, IASSID) was held in Washington, DC. The Association=s president, Professor Alan Clarke, commenting on the early origins of AAMD suggested that,

> ... a crude social Darwinism was often apparent, and correlates were usually mistaken for causes. An over-simple genetic and eugenic theory seems to have haunted the field. And in so far as environmental factors were thought to be etiologically relevant, parental tuberculosis and alcoholism were accorded prime importance" (1977, p.7).

Clarke went on to paint a more optimistic picture for the impact of human science from about the 1930s, indicating that organizations such as AAMD began to do more than reflect the social and political attitudes of the times.

Significant advances in scientific enquiry into intellectual disabilities were made in bio-medical and the growing social-behavioural disciplines in the pre- and post-World War II era on both sides of the Atlantic. However, for a variety of reasons, much of this work was conducted by scientists in relative isolation from each other.

The Birth of IASSMD

From its birth at the international meeting of scientists and administrators held in Copenhagen in 1964, and led by the late Harvey Stevens from the U.S.A. (a president of AAMD) and the late Alexander Shapiro from the U.K., IASSID has had a modest, yet growing, role in facilitating an exchange of scientific knowledge across national boundaries. In his insightful history of the Association, its first Secretary-General, Alan Clarke (1991) highlighted a number of factors which accelerated scientific enquiry in our field in the post war years. These included the spirit of optimism and humanism which attracted people to be more aware of disadvantage and to seek preventive or remedial measures. There was also a widespread belief that scientific methodology had much to offer. Of significance, too, was the strong growth of the parent lobby groups which impacted on policy and service provision at both national and international levels. Clarke also highlighted the impact of developments in the field of molecular biology, such as Lejeune's discovery of the extra chromosome in people with Down syndrome and the subsequent growth of the field of genetic counselling.

The late 1950s and early 1960s was also marked by the growth of the multidisciplinary nature of scientific enquiry in our field. Despite the broadening of the research base, much of the published work in these years followed a traditional functionalist, objectivist and positivist paradigm. Subsequent years, however, have seen the growth of new research paradigms which complement the traditional methodologies.

In its early years, the major means for facilitating the exchange of scientific endeavours used by the Association was the conduct of research-focused World Congresses, the first of which was held in Montpellier, France in 1967. Subsequent congresses were held in Warsaw, Poland (1970), The Hague, The Netherlands (1973), Washington, USA (1976), Jerusalem, Israel (1979), Toronto, Canada (1982), New Delhi, India (1985), Dublin, Ireland (1988), Gold Coast, Australia (1992) and Helsinki, Finland (1996).

During the relatively short history of IASSID since it foundation in 1964, the world has undergone remarkable socio-cultural, technological, economic and political changes which have impacted upon the lives of all, including people with disabilities. The pace of these changes has been almost exponential and great benefits have ensued for people generally.

Socio-cultural changes have resulted in a clear acknowledgment of the need for basic human rights for all. In many countries cultural diversity is being celebrated, but ethnic and religious divisions are still a depressing feature in both developed and developing countries. Of the massive technological advances, developments in communication must be among the most significant. The globalization of the world's economies has been starkly revealed by recent developments in Asia and the strong economic imperatives driving the unification of Europe. Possibly the most striking development, however, has been the growth of democratization across the world. Despite the continued presence of repressive regimes, strong democratic movements are emerging in Eastern Europe, Asia, Africa and South America.

These developments hold both positive and negative portents for people with intellectual disabilities. We have witnessed the impact of catalysts such as the normalization principle, the independent living and inclusion movements and more recently the empowerment of people with disabilities. However, these forces have had their greatest impact in countries experiencing sound economic growth and a parallel commitment to social justice. Significant legislative initiatives in the Nordic countries, Canada, USA and Australia, to name a few, occurred during periods of strong economic growth. With economic downturn and a subsequent move towards managerial economics there has been a striking weakening of political resolve to honor legislative statutes. A commitment to human rights and social justice without a concomitant fiscal policy puts the achievement of those rights at risk.

The last four decades have seen dramatic developments in all aspects of human endeavour. To keep pace with these changes IASSID has responded with changes in its structures. These have included changes in nomenclature with Amental deficiency being replaced with intellectual disabilities; the establishment of the category of subscribing individual members; the development of Regional Groups; and the adoption of the *Journal of Intellectual Disability Research* as the Association's official journal. Another major initiative has been the development of a number of Special Interest Research Groups (SIRGs). Congresses have also moved to a four-yearly cycle to complement the four-yearly cycle of Congresses of Inclusions International, our sister organization, which owes much to the energies and inspirational leadership of Gunnar and Rosemary Dybwad.

In the late 1960s IASSMD had collaborated with the then International League of Societies for the Mentally Handicapped (now INCLUSION INTERNATIONAL) to establish a Joint Commission on International Aspects of Mental Retardation under the auspices of the World Health Organization (WHO). The joint Commission with four members from each body has published a number of position papers including the problems of people with intellectual disabilities in the developing world and principles of assessment of intellectual disability. It also encouraged preventive programs such as iodine supplementation and the WHO Expanding Program for Immunization for all children.

At the Tenth Congress held in Helsinki in 1996, Council resolved to recommend to WHO the suspension of the Joint Commission, with each organization seeking independent status as a Non-Government Organization with WHO. In achieving this status IASSID has entered into an agreement with WHO to develop a number of position papers to be presented at its Eleventh Congress to be held in Seattle, USA, in August, 2000. The responsibilities for the development of these papers rest with a number of the SIRGs including Aging, Physical Health, Mental Health and Quality of Life.

These recent initiatives have had the effect of maintaining a momentum of international activities between the regular Congresses. They are also assisting in the pursuance of relevant research topics which involve a range of disciplines and a variety of scientific paradigms. Of particular note they are involving many more scientists in the ongoing activities of the Association. The development of Regional Groups will enable issues peculiar to a region to be explored.

The Association has not been noted for its involvement in political action, with one striking exception. Its Executive took a strong stand in 1970 when the Communist regime in Poland removed Dr Ignacy Wald from the Chairmanship of the Local Organizing Committee for the Warsaw Congress and attempted to prevent his acceptance of the position of Honorary Vice President of the Association. Dr Wald had been an outspoken critic of the Warsaw Pact's invasion of Czechoslovakia.

Scientists in our field must play a more active role in advocating for people with disabilities, especially in supporting the various human rights initiatives of the United Nations. In particular, we need to join with colleagues in the disability field who are supporting the initiatives of the *Standard Rules for the Equalization of Opportunities for Persons with a Disability*. In this respect, research has an important role to play (Parmenter, 1997a). Various human rights declarations indicate the goals for people with disabilities, but the processes and the outcomes of these initiatives are seldom tested. Do people with disabilities in countries which subscribe to the spirit of human rights principles in fact achieve an equalization of opportunity in their life domains?

Trends in International Research

It would be interesting to compare the range and relative emphases of research topics presented at the Fourth World Congress of IASSID in 1976 to a data base of international research in 1996, including presentations at the Tenth World Congress of IASSID (Parmenter, 1997b).

THE 1976 CONGRESS OF IASSID

A total of 481 presentations were made to the Washington Congress which the Association's editor, Peter Mittler (1977) classified into the categories of Care and Intervention; Education and Training; and Biomedical Aspects. Seventy-two percent of the presentations fell into the former two categories (36% each) with 28% in the Biomedical Aspects. Topics under Care and Intervention included research on policy, attitudinal studies, ethical issues, epidemiology, early intervention, families, residential services, community living, psychiatric services and cost-effectiveness studies. Within Education and Training topics included assessment, cognition and learning, adaptive behaviour, language and communication, educational and behavioral intervention, vocational rehabilitation and computer assisted instruction. The Biomedical Aspects included diagnosis and screening, genetic disorders, inborn errors of metabolism, prevention and treatment, environmental hazards, toxic origins, malnutrition, neuroscience and neuropsychological aspects.

One of the strong themes in the 1976 Congress was prevention. The breakthroughs in the identification of chromosomal abnormalities since the late 1950s were the focus of attention and there was expressed optimism that routine maternal screening and other biomedical advances would relieve the incidence of the severe grades of intellectual disability. There was also a growing awareness of the role environmental toxins played in causing neurological defects.

The Congress also reflected advances in educational programs that were able to raise the performance levels of persons with an intellectual disability, although questions were asked concerning the extent to which these advances were widely applied in the field. There was concern that many practitioners were consistently underestimating the potential of the people they worked with and low expectations were associated with poor provision and the subsequently poor outcomes.

In the area of the milder forms of intellectual disability the research findings of Edgerton and Bercovici (1976) and Cobb (1972) had a considerable impact. This work indicated that a high proportion of adults with mild intellectual disabilities achieved satisfactory adjustments. However, serious concerns were expressed about the growing gap between research and practice. Clarke (1977) in his presidential address commented,

> A few centres and a few institutions are doing excellent work, and using to the full our new knowledge. But where substantial new resources have been offered, authorities have been more bewitched by the need for splendid new buildings rather than by planning splendid new programs.... In the main our practice is based on a model of man that research has completely overturned. (p. 16, 17).

The Congress theme, "Research to Practice in Mental Retardation," was therefore quite apposite.

The problems faced in developing countries were alluded to but gained little attention in the overall program. The hope was expressed that the World Health Organization (WHO) might be able to play a key role in the prevention and amelioration of intellectual disabilities.

In keeping with the Congress theme a call was made for the more rigorous testing of the ecological and external validity of much of the published research. Commentators noted, too, the imbalance between pure and applied research, with the latter apparently being less valued. It was suggested that more field-based real life experiments were needed.

Other issues which emerged included the problem of definition. The Program Chair, Michael Begab, in his closing address drew attention to the lack of consistency in applying a definition which included both intellectual and behavioral criteria. There was a widespread failure to include adaptive behavior measures for diagnostic, placement or research purposes. Begab (1997) also highlighted the growing polarity of thought between those who saw intellectual disability as a relative, dynamic condition, varying as a function of particular settings and those who adopted a clinical perspective of intelligence which is independent of social settings.

The debate between mainstream and segregated services for this population, especially in the area of special education, was also evident with questions being raised concerning the methodological weaknesses of many of the comparison studies. In the area of living arrangements Begab noted that, despite the establishment of half-way houses, group care homes and an increased use of foster family care, there has been no systematic effort to determine what factors within those various settings are most contributory to successful placement....Evaluation of recently initiated programs and experimentation with new models of care are essential if we are to avoid mistakes similar to those of the past in the institutional field (p.24).

Other areas identified for increased research efforts included genetic disorders, socio-environmental retardation, communication disorders and causes related to prematurity, low birth weight, and malnutrition. Clarke (1977) aptly summed up the thrust of the 1976 Congress by remarking that, the task of science (is) to reveal the ways in which our biological and social pathologies can be alleviated, and it is our task as scientists to see that these findings are widely disseminated and used with profit (p.17).

RESEARCH EFFORTS IN 1996

What is the picture 20 years later? In many respects the research topic areas are similar. What is significant is the spectacular growth of research efforts. Several new journals devoted to the field of intellectual disabilities have appeared; and increased travel and communication opportunities have allowed for cross-cultural exchange and collaboration.

The following data provide an international snapshot of the range of research topics reported in journals and conference proceedings in 1996. There are a number of caveats regarding the comprehensiveness and categorization of the data. First, not all international publications or conferences have been accessed, although the data reported are reasonably representative. Second, while the categorization may appear arbitrary, an effort was made to place a paper in what appeared to be the most logical topic area. The reporting of a category "research paradigms" is possibly the most debatable. However, given the increasing growth in the variety of methodological approaches to studying various aspects of intellectual disabilities it was felt such a category would highlight this diversity.

The data base consists of 1515 individual journal/conference papers; 1048 presented to the 10th World Congress of IASSID in Helsinki, July, 1996; 375 published in 16 international journals, and 92 presented to a joint National Council of Intellectual Disability/Australia Society for the Study of Intellectual Disability held in Australia in 1996. Three key words were coded for each presentation, which allowed for up to three choices for a specific classification of the paper's major content focus. For instance, a paper classified into the aging category had dementia, mental illness and chronic physical problems as its key words. It would have been possible to place this paper in either the aging, mental health or physical health categories, but the major thrust of the paper was aging among people with an intellectual disability.

An examination of Figure 1 on the next page reveals the relative strength of research interests across the chosen seventeen categories. Papers with a major focus on policy issues, cognition, physical and mental health, and the diversity of research approaches, represented over 50% of presentations. Other topics with a strong representation were employment, family issues, education, genetics, quality of life and neurology. The topics advocacy, aging, ethics, gender, and legal issues, while among those with lower frequencies are, nevertheless, likely to be growth areas of research in subsequent years.

It is interesting that a division between biomedical and social/behavioral research indicates a 37% to 63% split. However, this relative bias towards social/behavioral research is possibly confounded by the fact that broad-based national and international conferences usually attract more presenters in this field than in the basic sciences. Likewise, the majority of journals accessed would tend to publish more research in the social/behavioral field than in the biomedical. Researchers in the latter field tend to report their results in discipline-based publications.

However, the growing diversity of research interests and research paradigms reflect significant developments in our field. These trends certainly support the predications made by Rowitz in 1992, particularly the following as higher frequency interest: changing paradigms of disability, quality of life, families and family care giving across the life span, aging; prevention and genetic breakthroughs, mental illness and intellectual disability, health care, supported living and employment models, legal issues, data bases and policy issues, and meeting more needs with less resources (Rowitz, 1992).

In comparing the emphases of research in the 1970s with that 20 years later, a number of issues are worthy of comment. Possibly one of the most significant developments is the way contemporary models of disability are influencing the research questions that are being asked, and the use of emerging scientific paradigms to explore the answers. Marcia Rioux (1997) in her keynote presentation to the Tenth World Congress in Helsinki commented,

> ways of viewing disability, of developing research questions, of interpreting research results, of justifying research methodology and of putting policies and programs in place are as much about ideology as they are about fact (p.102).

Rioux drew attention to the two very different world views of the nature of society alluded earlier to by Mercer (1992), who in turn referenced the work by Burrell and Morgan (1979) on sociological paradigms and organizational analysis. One view of society is centralizing and homogenizing, while the opposite stresses difference and diversity. Another dimension concerns the nature of reality, with objectivism and subjectivism being at opposite poles. Mercer has contrasted the two realities by suggesting that the objective view is external to the individual, and is hard, measurable, predictable and universalistic in meaning while the subjective

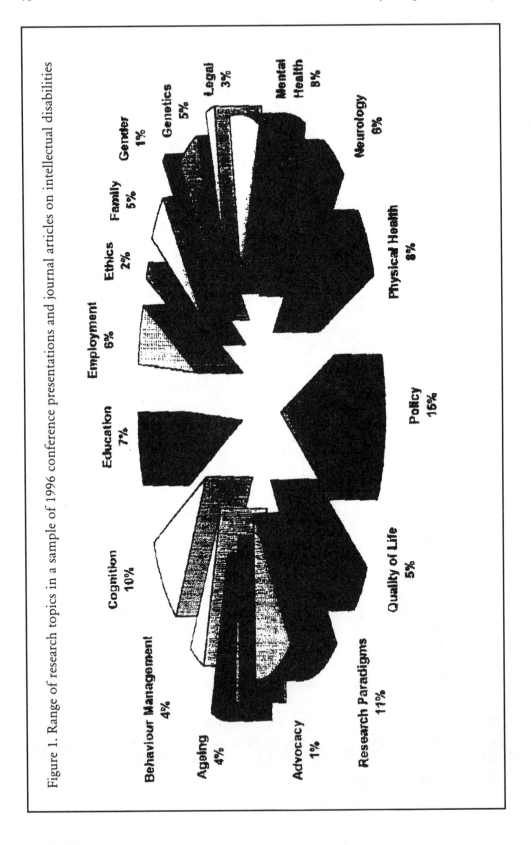

Figure 1. Range of research topics in a sample of 1996 conference presentations and journal articles on intellectual disabilities

view emphasizes the fact that human cognition is the crucial screen through which all experience is interpreted (p.17).

It would appear that over the 20 years this analysis has been made, the division between the biomedical and social/behavioral streams of research has been maintained. Of significance, however, is the growing diversity of methodologies used, especially in the latter area. The functionalist-objectivist paradigm which combined the homogeneous view of society with the objectivist view of reality had formerly dominated both streams of research. An area of research which is increasingly seeing a more interpretative paradigm in both the streams is investigations into quality of life. Here both the subjective-objective dimensions of reality must be recognized.

A related field is the increasing attention being given to ethical issues, especially those related to prevention. New discoveries emerging from the human genome project present a range of ethical issues that are being addressed by both scientists and consumer groups such as Inclusion International. On the one hand, there is the view that the possibilities offered by genetic advances will bring about a new eugenics movement offering increasing choices in human reproduction which question the essential nature of our human existence. The age of the "designer" baby may be upon us. Opponents to these developments are concerned that diversity in the human condition is being jeopardized by the uncritical embracing of these new discoveries. There is the counter argument that these scientific advances will ameliorate or prevent many of the diseases which reduce the potential for life quality for many people. It is suggested that like other major discoveries in the health field, for instance, penicillin, it will lead to spectacular improvements in the health and well being of the population.

A mechanism where IASSID is playing a role is in encouraging informed debate through its SIRG on Ethics. We should be encouraging researchers to engage in the social, philosophical and moral debates, for the implications of the genome project surely transcend the level of molecular biology.

There are signs, too, that an increasing emphasis upon studying the interaction of the individual with his/her environment may become a mechanism to unite the biomedical and social/behavioral streams of research. Early research, and much of that reported in the 1970s, still concentrated primarily on the individual and his/her limitations. In the social/behavioral field the 1970s saw an emphasis on programs to improve the competencies of the person with an intellectual disability. While competencies are still a focus, there is an increasing trend towards an examination of environmental supports that will reduce handicap and facilitate greater participation of the person in his/her community (Verdugo, 1997). The 1992 Revision of the *Definition and Classification of Mental Retardation* (AAMR, 1992) and the current Revision of the *International Classification of Impairment, Activities and Participation (ICIDH-2)* by the World Health Organization (WHO, 1997), both reflect a growing appreciation of the environmental context and the emerging social paradigm of disability.

Disappointingly, the last 20 years have not seen a dramatic increase in the numbers of longitudinal studies which can illuminate the long-term effect of programs and social policies on the lives of people with an intellectual disability. A striking parallel, however, to the work of Edgerton (1967, 1976) in the USA has been the recently published work of Stephen Richardson and colleagues (Richardson & Koller, 1996), concerning the lives of intellectually disabled people in Scotland. Obtaining funding for this type of research, and finding people with the persistence of Edgerton and Richardson, are key factors in determining growth in this field of endeavour.

One must also echo the words of Michael Begab cited above. There is still a dearth of studies which actually examine the processes of achieving desirable program outcomes. Why do some school inclusion programs work better than others? Why are some community living programs not delivering good quality of life outcomes? While we may have moved from a preoccupation with buildings, as alluded to by Alan Clarke, we are still, to some extent, locked psychologically into the deinstitutionalization phase of program development. Despite the fact that there still are large numbers of people in large congregate care environments, we must acknowledge that most people with intellectual disabilities across the world have never lived in such environments. We need to take a more proactive, rather than reactive approach to the issues on which we need to focus our research questions.

CHALLENGES FOR THE NEXT MILLENNIUM

In the context of the socio-cultural, technological, economic and political trends which will accompany us into the next millennium, scientists have a vital role to play in ensuring that people with an intellectual disability continue to see improvements in their quality of life. While discipline-based research will continue independently, IASSID has the challenge to assist in the co-ordination of research and application of its findings so that we do not lose sight of the whole person with an intellectual disability.

A recurring theme of our Congresses has been "research to practice". However, we need to address how research, policy and practice can be better integrated. As scientists we have often been too remote from the lives of the people we are studying. We have not included them nor their families and carers sufficiently well into our research planning. We have also been reluctant to engage in debates in the political arena. Concluding remarks by Victor Wahlström, a Past President of Inclusion International, in his presentation to the Helsinki Congress in 1996, provides us with salutary challenges. Victor posed the following questions:

1. What can your organization and the professionals do to make your research more operative, to make your research come to be used? For doing that you will need policy decisions leading to action.

2. What can your organization do to make your research known and used by persons with an intellectual disability and their families? To do that you need to present your research in a simple way and spread it.
3. What can you do to encourage the professionals to promote human rights even more forcefully to be watchdogs of the rights of persons with intellectual disabilities and never ever close ranks?

As scientists we cannot ignore these challenges.

Competition for resources will prove to be keener in the coming decades. Indeed, equity in resource allocation, exacerbated by neo-liberal economic philosophies, will prove to be one of the major ethical issues the world will face. The aging population in all countries will, it is predicted, place heavy welfare demands upon the decreasing work force. How will disadvantaged groups fare in economic environments that are currently increasing the gap between the elite "haves" and the dispossessed "have nots"? Depressingly, the same gaps are appearing in developing countries, where the majority of people with an intellectual disability are to be found. Have we lost the spirit of optimism and humanism alluded to earlier by Alan Clarke? It is therefore important for us to be more active in our advocacy role, joining with other international bodies to assist in keeping the needs of our population high on the political agendas.

As we move into the next millennium, we need to reach out more to developing countries. The origins of IASSID were essentially influenced by North American and Western European researchers, who still dominate its activities. Despite its limited resources the Association has a duty to encourage and support indigenous research efforts. We especially need to be cautious in applying Western delivery systems to cultures which have different histories and mores. We also need to listen to, and observe, how other cultures solve their own problems. As the days of relatively generous resources may be gone for us in the developed world, we, in the West, may learn how to effect advances in the life quality of people with intellectual disabilities using simpler and less costly means.

Reflection upon the advances we have made over the past century in philosophies, practices and research in the field of intellectual disability provide us with a degree of satisfaction that much has been accomplished that has enriched the lives of people with intellectual disability, their families, and the community generally. Just as we have supported inclusive public policies, the time may have come for researchers to reach out more actively into the generic fields of the research community. Have we been too insular in our research endeavours? Have we concentrated too much upon a pathology mentality? How do we reconcile our continuing search for prevention, while at the same time valuing the lives of people with existing disabilities? Studying the rich array of diversity in the human condition in the wider community may help us all realise that to be different is normal. Finally, as Rioux (1997) exhorts us, we must recognize the influence our judgments concerning the nature of disability have upon the way we study and interpret the "facts" of our research.

References

American Association on Mental Retardation (AAMR) (1992). *Mental Retardation. Definition, classification, and systems of support.* 9th Ed. Washington, DC: Author

Begab, M.J. (1977) Some priorities for research in mental retardation. In P. Mittler (Ed.). *Research to practice in mental retardation. Proceedings of the fourth congress of the International Association for the Scientific Study of Mental Deficiency.* Volume 1, A21-A30.

Burrell, G. & Morgan, G. (1979) *Sociological paradigms and organizational analysis.* Portsmouth, N.H.: Heinemann.

Clarke, A.D.B. (1977) From research to practice. In P. Mittler (Ed.). *Research to practice in mental retardation. Proceedings of the Fourth Congress of the International Association for the Scientific Study of Mental Deficiency.* Volume 1, A7-A19. Baltimore: University Park Press.

Clarke, A.D.B. (1991) A brief history of the International Association for the Scientific Study of Mental Deficiency (IASSMD). *Journal of Mental Deficiency Research,* 35, 1-12.

Cobb, H.V. (1972) *The forecast of fulfilment.* New York: Teachers College Press, Columbia University.

Edgerton, R.B. (1967) *The cloak of competence. Stigma in the lives of the mentally retarded.* Berkeley, CA: University of California.

Edgerton, R.B. & Bercovici, S.M. (1976) The cloak of competence: Years later. *American Journal of Mental Deficiency,* 80, 485-497.

Itard, J.M.G. (1962) *The wild boy of Aveyron.* New York: Appleton-Century Crofts.

Jull, K.D. (1981) Special education in Europe. In J.M. Kauffman & D.P. Hallahan (Eds.) *Handbook of special education.* Englewood Cliffs: Prentice Hall, 24-46.

Mercer, J.R. (1992) The impact of changing paradigms of disability on mental retardation in the Year 2000. In L. Rowitz (Ed.) *Mental retardation in the year 2000.* New York: Springer-Verlag, 15-38.

Mittler, P. (1977) (Ed.) *Research to practice in mental retardation. Proceedings of the Fourth Congress of the International Association for the Scientific Study of Mental Deficiency, Vols I, II, III.* Baltimore: University Park Press.

Parmenter, T.R. (1997a) Paper presented to K97 Human Rights for Persons with Mental Handicaps. Prague, Czech Republic.

Parmenter, T.R. (1997b) Paradigmatic shifts in scientific enquiry into intellectual disabilities. Evolution or revolution? Keynote address to Annual Conference of the Australian Society for the Study of Intellectual Disability. Brisbane, Australia.

Rioux, M. (1997) Disability: The place of judgement in a world of fact. *Journal of Intellectual Disability Research,* 41, 102-111..

Rowitz, L. (1992) Mental retardation in the year 2000. Prologue. In L.Rowitz (Ed.) *Mental retardation in the year 2000.* New York: Springer-Verlag, 3-11.

Richardson, S. & Koller, H. (1996) *Twenty-two years causes and consequences of mental retardation.* Cambridge: Harvard University Press.

Verdugo, M.A. (1997) Research on mental retardation: A priority agenda for the future. Keynote address to 121st Annual Meeting of the American Association on Mental Retardation, New York, USA.

World Health Organization (WHO) (1997) *International classification of impairments, activities, and participation.* Geneva: Author

3

Architectural Trends and Values
From Humanizing Institutions to Inclusive Communities

Elaine Ostroff
Adaptive Environments Center, Boston, MA

In 1966, Gunnar Dybwad convened an international meeting of architects in Copenhagen to consider the role of architects and how they might address the inhumane facilities in which people with mental retardation lived. That meeting was unique both in calling attention to the need for the involvement of the architect as part of the team as well as refocusing attention to the residents of the building. Dybwad urged the participants to focus on the residents and their needs, rather than administrative convenience. This chapter highlights a few of the ways in which the critical themes of people/environment interaction that Dybwad stressed at the Copenhagen conference have developed over time. They are all essential components in the creation of inclusive communities. They include the changing role of the architect and other designers as critical players in the planning team and the changing role of staff and consumers in the design of environments. Much of this work was initially supported by the Massachusetts Department of Mental Health. In addition, we introduce the concept of universal design, and describe the far reaching civil rights legislation in the United States that extended accessibility requirements into most of the built environment. Finally we detail a pilot program that addresses the challenge of educating future designers to meet the needs of a diverse society.

INTERNATIONAL WORKING CONFERENCE ON MENTAL RETARDATION

The International Working Conference on Mental Retardation was held in Copenhagen April 1966, co-sponsored by the Mental Retardation Project of the

---

Project Sponsors: The project would not have been possible without the following government and private foundations and organizations. They are: National Endowment for the Arts; US Department of Justice, Disability Rights Section; NEC Foundation of America; NYNEX Company; JM Foundation; and the Center for Universal Design.

International Union for Child Welfare and the Danish Mental Retardation Services. Gunnar Dybwad initiated the historic meeting in which 50 people, architects, administrators and practitioners from various countries, participated. The meeting marked the first public expression of both the problems with dehumanizing facilities as well as the significant role that the built environment and architects can have in the education and habilitation of people with mental retardation. In his introductory remarks Dybwad noted his growing appreciation of architects. Although he had visited more than 500 institutions over the previous 25 years, it was during his visit to Lillemosegaard in Copenhagen "'that he was struck with the tremendous contribution architects can make in our field". He made the strong connection between the growing awareness of the human potential of people with the most severely handicapping conditions and the need to express these values in concrete form. He explained,

> While the architect is in no position to control the activities of the institution or treatment center once it is built, he can create a physical setting which at the very least creates a natural setting for individualized treatment and normal patterns of living (unpublished remarks, 1966).

As always, Dybwad's talk pointed out the similarities in the environmental needs we all have as he noted the conference participants' grumbling about their conference accommodations for toilets and washrooms, and "even in new facilities, the remnants of the past, the toilets and facilities for washing and bathing that favored old impersonal institutional routines". Karl Grunewald, a child psychiatrist, head of the Swedish Mental Retardation Services and another speaker stated, "The basic difference between the past and the present is the overprotective and custodial care of the past versus the activating and outward looking care of today." He added, "The architectural design and layout of a building and its surroundings can either restrict further development or serve as the outer framework for a progression" (Dybwad, 1970). Dybwad pushed further, as to the location, and number and type of facilities. He invited the architect's knowledge of building design and materials to contribute to the choices.

In describing the meeting Dybwad reported, "There was great influence from the direct exchange of opinions, without any disturbing communication from the outside world.... It was an exciting meeting because of the many innovative ideas we exchanged of ways how the traditional forms of institutional design could be humanized to create dynamic space for living and learning".

He hoped the exchange would be followed by international action and it was. There were several important outcomes. Immediately, it led to changes in the design and construction of facilities in two countries. "One of the Yugoslavian architects wrote that upon his return he succeeded in canceling all their plans and that they are starting in with a totally different design on the basis of what he learned at our meeting. A government architect from Australia wrote: 'A major result from my attendance has been the re-planning of the patient's accommodation in our proposed Training Centers." (unpublished letter, Dybwad, 1966)

CHANGING THE ROLE OF THE ARCHITECT: THE DESIGNER AS FACILITATOR

In 1971, Elaine Ostroff's work at the Massachusetts Department of Mental Health, Division of Mental Retardation began a related approach to the problem of inhumane environments. Her process was through staff development, teaching classroom teachers and institutional staff as well as parents, how they could transform the environments in which they worked and lived. She named the process in which the designer taught their planning process to the users of the environment "Design Facilitation" (Ostroff, 1976).

As Coordinator of in-service Education for the Community Clinical Nursery Schools, she had the opportunity to visit most of the 100 classrooms of the statewide program. The compromising environments in which much of the teaching occurred were not the extremes of barren institutional places but rather the church basement, shared space situations common to many community programs for children with disabilities. She was struck at how the teachers accepted the poor learning environments as a given, and were unaware that they could make a difference both in the environment and in the children's ability through their collective effort. Her in-service education and technical assistance began a transformative process that the teachers could manage. She used a simplified space planning process that built on the knowledge the teachers had about their students. With recycled materials and a behaviorally based process that added environmental objectives to educational objectives, the teachers succeeded in making immediate improvements in their classrooms. There were two immediate benefits: the children were able to be more independent in an environment that facilitated their abilities and the teachers then had higher expectations for their students as they witnessed their newly visible skills.

A grim institutional space showed more dramatic results. A pilot project at the Dever State School transformed a day room and the behavior of a dozen adolescent boys that "destroyed everything" and "had no potential." The "day room" was an institutional euphemism for a room in which people were locked in during the day. The institutional staff contributed to the planning of the redesign that was managed by a team of design facilitators from the department. The photographs documented the changing behavior and the ability of the boys to interact with each other and the environment. The staff was eager to spend time with the students. The almost immediate impact was the transfer of several of the "untouchable" students to other programs that had educational goals.

Her work with staff led to the development of a graduate program in which the ability to manage environmental change was a core competence. Teams of graduate students funded through the Department of Mental Health Multi-Disciplinary Training programs demonstrated their leadership in the creation of new community-based programs and spaces to address unmet needs. The first cohort was at the University of Massachusetts, Amherst and later cohorts were at the Massachusetts College of Art. Their practicum experiences included the transformation of a garage in a community residence for children into a challenging play environment; the creation of a therapeutic playspace for medically fragile children out of an unused dining room at a pediatric nursing home; and the design and construction of a transitional learning environment in a public school for children moving from a state institution (Ostroff, 1997).

ADAPTIVE ENVIRONMENTS

Adaptive Environments was founded as a non profit educational organization in 1978, under a Federal grant. The original purpose was to support the integration of children with disabilities into regular classrooms through environmental design. This was in response to new Federal legislation that mandated the rights of all children for education in the least restrictive environment. Center staff taught a design process to the users of the environment - the teachers, therapists and parents, helping them plan adaptations to the classroom that would better meet the needs of the diverse children. Adaptive Environments staff, design educators, worked as facilitators to empower the users to improve their own space plans. Over the years, the mission became much broader, to create universally designed communities that support the participation of all people through education and advocacy for the civil rights of people with disabilities. Adaptive Environments is a small organization and has brought together teams of people to create national and regional programs. In all of the programs, people with disabilities play a significant role. More than half of the board of directors are people with disabilities.

UNIVERSAL DESIGN

This term is what we use in the United States to describe design that is usable by most people throughout their life span. We believe that universal design is design that goes beyond the technical requirements that are part of accessibility codes and standards. Ron Mace defined universal design as an approach to design that incorporates products as well as building features and elements which, to the greatest extent possible, can be used by everyone (Mace, 1988). It uses these standards as a base and encompasses the needs of people of all ages and abilities. The term "barrier-free" is used in the US as a limited term to signify code compliance. Some Europeans and the Japanese use that term in the broader sense. The concept that we share, if not the terminology, is thoughtful design, integral to the basic design, and not an add-on or an adaptation. It is good design. Universal design is often simple and invisible, it does not stand out. When describing a project that incorporates universal design it is usually necessary to explain how it meets the needs of many people, as it is not obvious.

There is a receptivity to universal design in the United States that began to be evident about seven years ago. There are two overall factors: the rapidly changing demographics and the far reaching civil rights laws that encompass much of the built environment.

The aging of our society has everyone's attention. Never before have there been so many people with such a long life expectancy. This growing population will not be living in nursing homes or institutions. We don't want to, we prefer to age in place, in our own community or in another community of choice. It also is impossible to build the numbers of new settings that would be required to house this remarkable aging population. There are stunning implications as we consider the changes needed in our communities to accommodate this changing social picture, especially as we acknowledge the physical and sensory changes that are a normal part of aging. This is a global issue - we hear the same concerns from other industrialized countries.

CIVIL RIGHTS LAWS AND ACCESSIBILITY

There are two recent Federal civil rights laws that include architectural access. They are the Fair Housing Amendments Act of 1988 and the Americans with Disabilities Act of 1990.

1. The Fair Housing Amendments Act, 1988. These amendments to the Fair Housing Act of 1968 were quite revolutionary. The Fair Housing Act of 1968 was passed to prohibit housing discrimination against people of color. With the 1988 amendments, people with disabilities and children were added as protected classes in relation to housing. For the first time in our history, the civil rights of people with disabilities would be addressed not only in programs or buildings that used federal funding but in privately funded housing. In passing this legislation, the government made it clear that the civil rights of people included a choice as to where they might live.

The legislation is very broad and deals with the rental and sale of residential properties as well as administrative policies. It also covers the modification of existing housing and introduces standards for the construction of new, multi-family dwellings with four or more units. The intent is to minimize stigmatizing, separate "handicapped" units that are often difficult to find or to rent. When a person needs an accessible unit, there may not be one where they would like to live. And, when a realtor is trying to rent an accessible unit to someone who may not immediately need the access, they react to the "handicapped look." The Fair Housing

Amendments Act (FHAA) Design Guidelines include seven requirements that introduce the basis of universal design in new construction. These are modest requirements and may not meet the needs of people with more severe needs. They do not replace the requirements for some percentage of fully accessible units, but they are creating choices for the future. They include 1) accessible exterior routes from transportation and parking, and accessible entrances; 2) accessible and usable common spaces; 3) all doors to allow passage by people who use wheelchairs; 4) an accessible route within each unit; 5) usable heights for electrical outlets and switches, 6) adaptable bathrooms and 7) usable kitchens.

2. Americans With Disabilities Act, (ADA) 1990. Only two years after the FHAA was passed, the ADA was passed with support from both political parties. Like the FHAA, this significant legislation was not limited to federally supported programs as did earlier civil rights legislation Section 504 of the 1973 Rehabilitation Act. It covers private, commercial businesses as well as all state and local programs. There are very few exemptions, one is for religious entities. There was a tremendous amount of cross disability advocacy across the country. It was a time of great coalition building with every organized group of people with disabilities. There was both a strong grass roots effort in every state throughout the nation as well as a well organized machine in the nation's capital in Washington, DC. People with disabilities were able to make a strong case for the right to work, to participate and to be contributors to society.

The ADA is often described as a "patchwork quilt" of legislation as it covers all the distinct areas where the other citizens had rights but where there was discrimination against people with disabilities. It provides equal opportunity in employment, private businesses, government services, public and private transportation and telecommunications. It is not an affirmative action law, giving preferences to people with disabilities; rather it mandates equal opportunity. The government was very clear that architectural barriers prevent equal opportunity and are a form of discrimination. The ADA is not only about architectural barriers. It includes communication access as well as facility access, and all of the ways that business and government work to make their services available to people as employees and as customers.

The ADA covers most facilities and addresses accessibility in a number of ways. It covers existing buildings as well as alterations and new construction. The arguments about existing buildings were finally resolved with a compromise. The two opposing views were:

a. All existing buildings should be made fully accessible, bringing them up to new construction standards;
b. Ignore existing buildings and only begin to remove barriers when an alteration project was begun.

The compromise created a new standard, "Readily Achievable" barrier removal. It established a process by which building owners, operators and managers could determine if it would be possible for them to remove some small barriers in ways that are cheap and easy. This was one of the most controversial aspects of the law and the one that got the most attention and created anxiety. Never before had there been requirements for existing buildings to achieve some level of access. Architects had become aware, if not competent, in following requirements when they had to make alterations or plan new construction; this was commonplace across the country. "Readily Achievable" was an extraordinary new challenge, one that required a measure of thinking, and would benefit from the participation of people with disabilities in setting priorities for barrier removal.

The ADA also created a uniform set of nationwide architectural standards that had to be followed for all alterations or new construction in commercial facilities. This was the ADA Standards for Accessible Design. It was in this spotlight of the FHAA, the ADA, with the heightened awareness of the design professions of regulations covering most of the built environment, along with the growing interest, concern and market potential of the aging society that we created the Universal Design Education Project.

UNIVERSAL DESIGN EDUCATION PROJECT

In 1989 we knew that the ADA was close to becoming law, and that this was the beginning of "the teachable moment" when we might capture the attention of design educators. There was much evidence that designers were not understanding what accessibility was all about. Although every state in the union had some accessibility standards for new construction, buildings were still being constructed with thoughtless barriers built in, or awkward code compliant solutions added late in the design process. The dominant attitudes of designers were reflected in a double standard of design – the "good" design as opposed to grudgingly compliant design. Universal design was considered a trendy euphemism for "handicapped design," and a specialized response for limited numbers of people in specialized settings.

We knew that future designers were not being educated to meet the needs of diverse users who may be unlike themselves. The recommendations made much earlier by a group of design practitioners and educators emphasized that we teach ways of designing that "go beyond the codes," toward universal design (Ostroff, 1982). What was needed was a broad based new approach to design education that would help change attitudes about who we are designing for. We had a strong model developed by Professor of Architecture Ray Lifchez from the University of California at Berkeley. He brought consultants, people with disabilities, into the design studio as a way for students to begin designing for people unlike themselves. There were many successes in the studio, and the work is well documented in the book *Rethinking Architecture* (Litchez, 1986) and in the video *A House for Someone Unlike Me* (Bassett, 1984).

We believed there were good teachers all the country who were teaching about accessibility. However, their work was often an add-on course, someone's pet topic, and not seen as central to the professional course of study. There was no coherent documentation of what was being taught nor any support for their innovations. Universal design, if the term was used at all, had different meanings for different people. With this awareness, we developed the Universal Design Education Project. The pilot program is documented in *Strategies for Teaching Universal Design* (Welch, 1995).

We describe it as a "grassroots, incentive approach." We wanted to stimulate creative teaching efforts to infuse universal design in many different design disciplines and schools. Each university, each department has its own culture. We believed for any innovation to take root it must come from the faculty, and that a top down approach, an imposed curriculum, would not be accepted. We created an awards program of stipends for faculty members who would submit proposals for curriculum projects that would begin to integrate universal design in the school curriculum. The approach should reflect the culture of each place and have some chance for continued development and institutionalization.

RECRUITMENT AND SELECTION PROCESS

We created a strong national advisory board, comprised of the leading practitioners and educators in universal design. This included Ron Mace, of the Center for Universal Design and one of the first proponents of the concept and the term. The advisors would be part of the peer review process in selecting the recipients of the stipends. We engaged the professional design education societies who helped promote the awards program and mailed announcements to each department chair in every design school in the country. The request for proposals was quite demanding. Faculty had to describe their proposed strategies, how it was integral to the overall curriculum, explain how they would document and evaluate their work, show support of the department and detail the ways in which people with disabilities would be involved.

We selected faculty from 22 schools for the first cycle of the program in 1993 - 1994. They included a total of 45 faculty members in architecture, industrial design, interior design, and landscape design. The second pilot, in 1995 - 1996, included nine schools and 27 faculty. Some schools were funded for a second time, so that a total of 25 schools and 60 faculty have participated in the project . They represent a mix of tenured and junior faculty, and both multi-disciplinary teams as well as single disciplines.

TECHNICAL ASSISTANCE TO FACULTY

The project supported the selected faculty in a number of ways. The initial colloquium was held at the Center for Universal Design at North Carolina State University. This intense meeting was the beginning of a strong network and a community of effort that would reinforce each person's individual work. There were multiple learning opportunities: presentations, so that all participants had a shared vocabulary and images; small work groups, interactive exercises and large group discussions and brainstorming.

1. Each school received a kit of teaching tools that consisted of a binder full of background materials with reproducible articles and video tapes. Most of the publications about universal design were displayed in a comprehensive book exhibit that invited browsers.
2. Each school had an advisor, someone from the national advisory group, who maintained contact with them through periodic telephone calls.
3. The advisors visited each school, making a major public presentation, met with deans and department chairs, with the faculty team and with students.
4. The project organizer, Adaptive Environments, maintained contact through periodic mailing of updates and new materials.
5. An Internet website, www.adaptenv.org was developed and became a repository for information about all of the programs.

RANGE OF TEACHING STRATEGIES DEVELOPED BY FACULTY

The faculty developed an extremely diverse range of teaching strategies. The 21 case studies in the book give much insight about what the faculty generated and the ways in which they tried to infuse universal design in the curriculum. It included broad based changes to existing seminars and studios, intensive design charrettes involving university wide participation computer assisted teaching modules, university wide courses and design competitions. Some faculty created a new elective but made links to other courses and studios.

The Role of User/Experts In the Process

The single most important teaching and learning technique involved user/experts. This is the term that we created to describe the consultants with disabilities, some older persons, and some younger persons, and people of extreme heights, who participated in most of the schools. We needed a term that would accurately reflect the contribution that each could make. Every person was an expert in their own experience with the environment. This, and their humanity, was what they were bringing to the students.

The faculty proposed many different and creative ways to engage users in the teaching and learning process; many were able to carry out their plans successfully. In some instances students with disabilities were enrolled in the design studio. In other schools, they arrived as surprise guest critics, shocking the unexpecting students. The methods that the faculty developed were as diverse as the schools themselves.

What Did We Learn?

1. The user/expert is the most valuable resource in universal design education. We learned this from exit interviews, written evaluations, reports of spontaneous comments from students and discussions with faculty. Students reported that the interactions "completely changed their understanding about who they were designing for." "I feel that I will be a very different designer now than if I did not have these experiences". Throughout the program, most of the students were enthusiastic in their expanded awareness, realizing that limitations in ability, and the extremes in size and strength are common aspects of human existence, especially as one ages.

In their new awareness, they were often outraged at the inadequate designs of buildings and products for handicapping conditions. The project achieved a major objective, to engage the creative imagination of future designers to be inclusive in their thinking, and to think beyond their own young and able bodies as they design. Students who have participated in the project say, "Why would I want to design something that limits people's freedom of choice?" "I understand that everyone has some unique needs that we must consider when we design." "Anything that I design will be universally accessible, not because of laws but because I want it that way." "Universal design is now part of my own ethics."

However, the faculty reported that the involvement of user/experts has complications. There are administrative and organizational concerns as well as process issues. The payment of the user/experts is also a continuing concern. While faculty want to provide some honoraria, these are not always available. Faculty have developed alternative methods to compensate for people's time. Also, there is more to learn about the most effective ways to involve the user/experts, when during the course sequence how many different perspectives should be include; and how to avoid burn-out in using the same people over and over again.

2. We confirmed the concerns that many of us had about the use of simulations. There was overall agreement that in and of themselves they provide a distorted view of any person's life experience. They leave a false impression about living with a disability, and preclude more thoughtful investigation about the varieties of human experience. If simulations are to be used, they should be conducted

under the direction of experienced leaders with disabilities and be followed by significant discussion.

3. The sense of community is very important for faculty, to know that they are not alone in their values, and that there are other faculty and practitioners who have similar beliefs as well as experience to share. This contributed to what many faculty said, "This has been among my most satisfying and exciting teaching experiences".

4. Righteousness is to be avoided. Often we get so deeply involved with our mission there is a tendency to see other people as the unenlightened. Faculty must attempt to find ways to build bridges and communication with other faculty.

5. Infusion within the curriculum helps integrate knowledge. Students must learn these principles and approaches as part of their overall professional development. Multiple, developmental learning opportunities are necessary throughout each year; this is not a single exposure or inoculation;

6. Additional, in-depth courses may be needed to supplement technical knowledge.

7. Expanded communication about what has been designed is needed. Students need to learn how to articulate what they have created through discussion and through annotations on drawings to convey the invisible qualities of universal design. Additional narrative description is needed for users with low or no vision to convey the visual information. More innovations are needed to find new ways of communication for people who cannot read drawings.

WHERE DO WE GO NEXT?

We're still very much at the beginning. This was a small project in a large country. There are many schools where this is not happening. With what we have done, there is more documentation still to be analyzed. Some faculty were more successful than others, beginning work that continues and deepens each year. Some departments in certain schools were much more open to the faculty experiments, others were much more resistant. Every school made a contribution to the improvement of design education so that it is more responsive to social and user needs.

There are so many factors relating to change that we are still evaluating the impact. We are in the midst of longer term evaluations, from the faculty and from the students who have graduated. We want to know what difference their education is making in their design work. We want to know if the faculty can continue this work without as much support from the project, and what they want to help them sustain their teaching of universal design. We know that we can learn from each other. We live in an increasingly global economy and can only solve these challenges with international cooperation.

References

Bassett, B.W., 1984. *A house for Someone Unlike Me*. National Center for a Barrieer Free Environment, Washington DC (video).

Dybwad, G., 1970. *Architecture's Role in Revitalizing the Feild of Mental Retardation*. Journal of Mental Subnormality Vol 16, No. 30 June 1970.

Lifchez, R., 1986. *Rethinking Architecture*. University of California Press, Berkeley, CA.

Mace, R., 1988. *Universal Design: Housing for the Lifespan of All People*. US Department of HUD, Washington DC.

Ostroff, E. and Tamashiro, R., 1976. *Transforming Institutions with Play, the Arts and Environmental Design*. Final Report, University of Massachusetts, Amherst, MA.

Ostroff, E. and Atkins, G., 1977. *Humanizing Evironments, A Primer*. World Guild and Department of Mental Health, Boston, MA.

Ostroff, E. and Iacofano, D., 1982. *Teaching Design for All People: State of the Art*. Adaptive Environments Center, Boston, MA.

Welch, P., 1995. *Strategies for Teaching Universal Design*. Adaptive Environments Center, Boston, MA.

4

The Metaphor of Mental Retardation
Rethinking Ability and Disability

Douglas Biklen
Center for Human Policy, Syracuse University

Creating a Context for Seeing Ability

Recently I conducted an observation in a first grade inclusive classroom in which I observed a teacher who had an ability to ignore extraneous behavior and to create the conditions necessary for a student with autism and a severe communication impairment to communicate effectively. My focus was on a 7 year old student with autism who could speak a few words, usually only in single words, and who I never heard saying a sentence, except if she was reading from text in front of her. In a class lesson we see the kinds of speech she produced which then can be compared to her typing and writing:

> Mrs. Castle (Cathy's teacher) wrote the word *robot* on the chalk board, with a long vowel sound over the first *o* and a short one over the second one. She asked the students if they knew what the word spelled. Seven students raised their hands. She called on one boy who said "Rowboat." She pointed out that this was close but that the sound of the second "o" was different and that it

---

This chapter is based on a presentation, *Creating the Context for Expression*, made to the conference: Autismo E Comunicazione Facilitata, Verona, 23 May, 1998.

The statements made by persons with disabilities are presented in **bold type**. Prior to their using facilitation, each of the people cited in this chapter was identified as autistic, retarded and unable to communicate in sentence level conversation or writing. Since learning to communicate with facilitation, several have participated in research studies in which their authorship has been confirmed; others have achieved independent typing; and all use words and produce sentence constructions that are distinctive. Perhaps most persuasive of all, their themes convey validity, for they bespeak experience with disability and with a society largely ignorant to that experience.

sounded like "ah." Another student identified the word as *robot*. Mrs. Castle then asked, "What's a robot?" Students volunteered various answers, including: "It's an enemy; You fight it;" "It's metal and they don't think;" Mrs. Castle asked, "Cath, what do you think this is?" Cathy spoke, "Mr. Robot." Mrs. Castle then asked, "Right and what do you think a robot is?" She responded, "Lunch." The teacher smiled at her answer and remarked, "You've been reading ahead. That will become clear to everyone in a few minutes!"

After the class discussion, the students got out their books and read a story entitled "Mr. Robot," about an animal that had purchased a robot that could serve lunch. As the class read the story aloud, Cathy followed along, placing her finger on the words as they were said. An instructional specialist asked her to read aloud, and she began to do so, but she read very softly and only when it was demanded of her.

Although Cathy could speak, her teachers generally had to structure their questions to get expected, albeit brief responses. For example, when Mrs. Castle showed the class a picture of Martin Luther King and Coretta Scott dressed in wedding clothes and asked Cathy what they were doing. Cathy said, "Making." The teacher said, "What are they doing, Cathy?" Another student said, "getting married." Cathy said, "Married." Later, Mrs. Castle asked Cathy how she thinks Martin Luther King must have felt when other kids his age would not play football with him because he was black and they were white. Cathy had been fidgeting, with legs stretched out around a desk leg, near the rug, with her face on the leg, trying to bite the bolt on the leg. She did not make any expression and did not say anything. Mrs. Castle said, "Cathy, how would you feel if your good friend Stephanie said she would not play with you?" Cathy made a sad face and said, "Sad." During that same lesson, Mrs. Castle showed a picture of a casket and asked Cathy what had happened. Cathy said, "He died."

Despite the fact that she did not converse with others in spoken sentences, other than brief commands, Cathy wrote and typed with no physical support. For spoken responses, her teacher learned how and when to structure opportunities for Cathy to make contributions to the class discussion. And she knew how to frame these events positively, drawing attention to Cathy's strengths in reading. In this chapter I will attempt to explore how facilitated communication is helping to create a context whereby individuals who have previously been unable to express themselves effectively can now do so.

Mental Retardation as Metaphor

In the July, 1997 issue of the *New England Journal of Medicine,* Rapin, a neuropsychiatrist and expert on autism wrote, "Approximately 75 percent of persons with autism are mentally retarded; their cognitive level is significantly associated with the severity of their autistic symptoms" (p. 99). This statement fairly represents the dominant view within the field of autism. Jacobson, Mulick, and Schwartz (1995), for example, reported in the *American Psychologist*, that "mental retardation of varying degrees occurs at extremely elevated rates among people with autism" (p. 757). The tendency of the field has been to equate speech and action with thinking ability. In this regard, Jacobson et. al concluded that:

> general delays or deficits in language function are closely related to general delays or deficits in intellectual development. A corollary to the third point is that the everyday facility with which people with autism or mental retardation use a language (e.g., spoken, written, or pictorial) is an accurate depiction of their ability to do so and that there is no clinically significant phenomenon that inhibits the overt production of communication and "masks" normative communication skills (i.e., actual production is representative of "internal" speech skill). This standpoint is firmly grounded in an immense psychological literature in cognitive development, social development, and both general cognitive and social problem solving by children and adolescents .... That there is a strong presumptive relationship, in general, between overt production and actual ability is a cornerstone of psychological assessment methodology, statistics, and psychometrics (p. 757).

Rapin appears to agree with this pessimistic view:

> Comprehension and the communicative use of speech and gesture are always deficient, at least in young children with autism. A compromised ability to decode the rapid acoustic stimuli that characterize speech results in the most devastating language disorder in autism; verbal auditory agnosia or word deafness. Children with verbal auditory agnosia understand little or no language; they therefore fail to acquire speech and may remain nonverbal (p. 97).

The essence of Jacobson et al.'s and Rapin's statements is that we measure intent, ability, and intelligence by what people say or do.

A somewhat more targeted, though certainly related, metaphor is that most people with autism lack a "theory of mind," characterized especially by an inability to "understand other people's different beliefs" (i.e., different from one's own; Baron-Cohen, 1996, p. 71). Rapin similarly finds that "poor insight into what others are thinking persists throughout life. Creativity is unusually limited" (p. 99).

Common to each of these theories about the relationship of mental retardation to autism is the fact that researchers have observed the actions of people with autism and have then hypothesized what their actions mean, concluding that it is *as* if the person with autism is retarded or lacks a theory of mind. But we are wont to ask what is it that we *know* when we see another's actions? Is it justifiable to presume that a perceived absence of evidence of complex thinking in fact means that there *is* no complex thinking? In short, how do you know what someone knows?

Research on Facilitated Communication: Unexpected Competence in People with Autism

Now the question before us is whether mental retardation is an actual condition that resides in people with autism, as Rapin, Jacobson, and others would have us believe, or is it instead a metaphor which is critiqued by each instance in which people with autism find an effective means of communication? Recent evidence drawn from research on facilitated communication and related studies suggest the latter.

Facilitated communication is a type of augmentative and alternative communication (AAC) for people who do not speak or whose speech is highly limited and disordered, and who cannot point reliably (Biklen & Cardinal, 1997; Crossley, 1994). The method has been used by people with autism, Down syndrome, cerebral palsy, pervasive developmental disorders, and other developmental disabilities (Crossley & Remington-Gumey, 1992; Biklen, 1993; Crossley & Mc Donald, 1984; and Crossley, 1994).

Facilitated communication involves developing communication skills through pointing with a partner e.g. typing or pointing at pictures or letters. The communication partner provides physical support e.g., holding the person's wrist or forearm during pointing, providing backward resistance as the person tries to move the arm forward to point, or merely a hand on the shoulder as the person points or types. Facilitated communication, leading to independence, does not begin with only physical support, but like all AAC methods, involves other forms of prompts and cues, including constant feedback of letters typed or pictures and letters pointed to, reminders to look at the target, verbal coaxing to start pointing or to stop pointing repeatedly at one target item, asking clarification questions (e.g. "I'm not sure what you mean by that, could you explain?"), and encouragement (e.g. "keep going, you're doing fine" or "go ahead, you can do it".)

Many studies designed to prove that the facilitated communication user is expressing his or her own ideas have failed to do that (Wheeler, Jacobson, Paglieri, and Schwartz, 1993; Eberlin, McConnachie, & Volpe, 1993). These and other studies have also demonstrated that many facilitated communication users are easily influenced in their typing by the facilitator. More recently, however, a number of studies *have* shown that people using this method can prove that they author the words typed. The largest study of facilitated communication to date, conducted in the California public schools (Cardinal, Hanson, & Wakeham, 1996), included over 3,800 trials, more than all other facilitated communication studies combined. Students classified as "severely disabled" were asked to spell randomly selected words that they were shown while their facilitator was out of the room. Unlike prior studies which had failed to authenticate the authorship of individuals using facilitation (e.g. Klewe, 1993; Regal et al., 1993; Smith et al., 199 ;Wheele et al., 1992), Cardinal et al. (1996) allowed participants to *practice* the test activity extensively — though not the actual words; they were asked to spell five words per session in three sessions per week. By the end of the six-week study, with facilitation, 74 percent of the students were able to correctly spell one or more of the words that had been shown to them by the tester while the facilitator was out of the room; half were able to spell at least two of the five words. On average, students reached their peak performance at this task after nine sessions; they were unable to achieve these performance levels without facilitation.

Other studies that have authenticated authorship by people using facilitation include, for example, a study in which individuals with autism and other disabilities were asked to play computer games while the facilitator's view of the computer screen was blocked (Olney, 1995); another study involving extensive practice of the test procedure, where the individual was able to accurately name pictures (Marcus and Shevin, 1997). Marcus succeeded in the type of picture naming task that all of the Wheeler et al. participants failed. In another study, individuals reported on videos and books they read while the facilitator was in a different room, giving 79 instances of authentic communication under the facilitator blind condition (Sheehan and Matuozzi, 1995). Baldac and Parsons (1997) reported individuals passed messages to a naive facilitator about pictures they observed.

One of only a handful of studies in which individuals were asked to produce sentence level communication that included information unknown to their facilitators, reported a person believed to be severely retarded learned to communicate with facilitation.

> Kenny was a 13.5 year old boy at the date of the first test trial. His developmental status independent of his performance with facilitated communication was characterized by a diagnosis of autism, severe mental retardation, and a history of seizures. His most recent formal psychological evaluation, performed when he was 10 years of age by a school psychologist, resulted in a Full-Scale IQ of 31 (36 month age equivalent) on the Stanford Binet Intelligence Scale.
>
> Kenny's verbal production at the time of the facilitated communication testing procedures was almost entirely echolalic, perseverative, and/or self stimulatory in nature (he would often repeat words such as "fishy-fishy" or "NBIS-NBIS" (the acronym of a local bank), with no apparent meaning attached to these utterances). He had fewer than 10 words that he occasionally used functionally (e.g. he would say "soup" when hungry, call out "daddy" when trying to gain adults' attention). (Weiss, Wagner, & Bauman, 1996, p. 221).

Researchers read him several moral stories while his facilitator was out of the room. When asked questions about the stories, he demonstrated intuitive thought, literacy skills, and an ability to think about what others are thinking.

In one story, two boys played with a ball in the house and broke a lamp. Kenny successfully described who was involved and what happened, and imagined that the father was forgiving. In another story, two children get a BB gun against their parents' wishes. They accidentally break a window. Kenny deduced that the mother in the story would be mad. In neither case does the story tell us exactly how the parents feel.

Had Kenny responded incorrectly through his limited echolalia or unreliable pointing, we would only be able to *interpret* what he knows. And we might easily misinterpret, taking his action as emblematic of his thoughts. Now that he has more elaborate communication, he escapes the ranks of the mentally retarded and gives evidence suggesting that he can intuit the feelings of others.

From these diverse studies, two things become clear. First, for people with autism who have significant communication impairments, the ability to reveal literacy, complex thoughts, and intelligent thinking depends greatly upon context. These include test conditions (Biklen and Cardinal, 1997; Dwyer, 1996), availability of and training in alternative means of communication (e.g. facilitated communication, typing), help with inhibiting impulsive responses, as well as personal knowledge or thinking ability. Related to this, in terms of testing literacy abilities, it is important to remember that a test must itself be valid for our intended purpose before we can rely on findings from it. The fact that a study appears quite simple from the perspective of a non-disabled person, does not make it simple to do for a person with autism or other developmental disability. And if the test inhibits performance that could reveal complex thinking abilities, then the test may be falsely interpreted to imply mental retardation. Simply put, not all tests *are* valid. And for people with autism, the task of developing sensitive tests that allow individuals to reveal themselves effectively, whether the tests purport to assess intelligence or something like facilitated communication, has often proved difficult indeed.

In those instances where people with autism have gained an effective means of communication, judgments of them being retarded seem to fall away. To ensure continued education, educators must learn to create contexts to maximize it.

Lessons From a Life: Breaking Through Mental Retardation

A number of individuals who first began to communicate with facilitation are now able to type without any physical support. And recently some individuals who use facilitation to type are able to read aloud what they type. Others have passed tests proving their communicative competence. In the section which follows I will examine my conversations with one individual who has *learned to read aloud what he types*

with facilitation. I will augment my analysis of his thoughts with those of other facilitated communication users who have in their own ways proven their communicative competence. And, as a further kind of triangulation of data and meaning, I will relate these accounts by people using facilitation with reports
from people with autism who communicate in conventional speech and writing and who have written autobiographies, including Williams (1994) and Barron (Barron and Barron, 1992). The main part of this section is drawn from my conversations with Richard Attfield. Finally, reflecting on what can be learned from individuals' experiences, I will suggest strategies for creating the context for effective communication and participation.

DESCRIPTION OF COMMUNICATION AND PRESUMED ABILITY/DISABILITY

Up until the age of 15, Richard attended special schools. His mother describes his curriculum as chiefly "life skills. They did targets, you know putting laundry in the machine, telling time, things like that." For exercise they did calisthenics:

> You probably know that with Richard you'd have to move his arms. When they were doing Mr. Motivator, Richard's worker was standing by his side doing it all, and Richard just standing there doing nothing. This was at a school that was supposed to be specialized.

Science was comprised of disjointed activities such as "seeing steam rise from the kettle." In the last years of his schooling, after his parents had started Richard on facilitated communication, the special school began to give Richard some academics, but when it was time for him to leave that school and transition to adult life, the psychologist referred him to a day center for people with mental retardation.

Richard was intent on a different future. Using facilitated communication, he wrote to a number of colleges and eventually found one to accept him. In his first year he took a course in art history and another in literature, studying Shakespeare, among others. And during this first year of college, Richard won a writing award and also developed his newfound ability to read aloud what he types.

Push me:
As if to assure that we not slip into stereotypical thinking about how to support people with disabilities in school, another autobiographer, Birger Sellin (1994), lets us know that he has boundless energy and needs above all people who will push him to greater levels of performance. Though his autism often leaves him blank looking, even seemingly frozen in inaction, not unlike Williams' student Jody above, inside he really does want to act, and needs his teachers' help. In the book, *I don't want to live inside me anymore,* Sellin has

written,
> *Which would you rather*
> *for me not to live(,) without help and stay handicapped*
> *or for me to become independent,*
> *if so you must just demand more from me.* (p. 184).

His words echo those of an expert in the education of students with autism, Rosalind Oppenheim who argues in her book, *Teaching Methods for Autistic Children and Youth*, that in every lesson, every day, the student should be given opportunities to try something on his or her own, independently. Oppenheim observes that the same student can be competent in one setting when pushed to perform and thoroughly incompetent in another when expected to fail. She describes a student who one year is observed making statistical calculations with ease and in another year seems incapable of the simplest addition calculation.

Sellin's account is also reminful of one involving another young autistic student, Ian, in Martin's book *Out of Silence* (1995), where Ian insists on having a new selection of foods and films, even though he shrieks and hits when given them. He tells his parents to be especially firm with him, that his actions do not reflect his desire, only that he reacts involuntarily and harshly to changes which threaten his obsessions of eating only a few foods and viewing only one or two films repetitively. His flailing body and his shrieks often are not indicative of a resistant person, only an anxious one.

In one inclusive school we had the experience of a young student with autism repeatedly running from the classroom during science and language arts instruction out onto the playground. His teachers tried to contain him, but he often fled to the playground when they were not looking. When we queried him, he said he really did understand that he should stay in the classroom, but that he sometimes felt compelled to run onto the playground. Fortunately, the student came up with an answer to the problem. He told his teachers to be firm with him and to place a sign on the door that said, "Do not leave the room without a teacher's permission." This sign was enough to help him stay and continue to participate in the science and language arts lessons.

Clearly facilitation is more than holding someone's arm and more than a technique to augment communication; it is also a strategy for fostering fuller participation in many aspects of daily living.

AWARENESS OF THE WORLD

In my conversations with Richard, I was interested in how he would interpret the types of situations about which people with autism are often presumed to be unaware. For example, I asked Richard about crossing streets. What did he think about the idea that a person with autism is typically presumed unable to recognize dangerous situations, such as an oncoming car.

"I guess I never have run out into the road," Richard typed.

Hearing this, his mother reminded him of an instance where he did just that: "how about the day you left school, what about that day?" She explained that he was on an outing with his class in the woods and he wanted a drink of water. When he was told he'd have to wait, he hid behind a tree and then ran away. His teachers later found him sitting outside a pub.

"I guess I ran across the road. But nothing hit me," Richard explained.

"Well what about this matter of dangerousness?" I asked.

"Okay I know that it is dangerous to run out in the road in front of cars. I guess I do not look at the busy road. I think how good it is to be freed from supervision. I think, great! No one to tell me what to do. Okay, I guess it has to be lack of experience. I guess I never expected to know how to cross a road. I am trying it."

(To help himself achieve it, he imagines that he is *not* alone.)

Richard presents an interesting perspective. On the one hand he says he has had a tendency to focus on one thing (e.g. being free) and not another (traffic).

Does this mean he could not be aware of traffic or that he is not aware of the world and its dangers? Does this suggest difficulties with attention shifting? Does it suggest, as Richard explains, lack of practice and experience with certain events? And along with his lack of practice, does he also have some trepidation about now doing it alone, so much so that he develops the coping strategy of imagining he is not alone? So can we surmise that anxiety affects performance and therefore perceptions of others about his understanding?

Richard's mother pointed out, during this conversation, that she sometimes saw the teenage students at Richard's school "coming out (of the school) with workers holding their hands, even students who were not physically disabled, students who could have walked by themselves." It was not until it became clear that Richard was going to go to college that the school agreed to work on that skill.

Best selling author Donna Williams (1994), in her second autobiographical account of autism, describes similar difficulties with performance, and she credits her own competing sensory functions, leaving her seemingly unconscious/not understanding side-by-side with excellent, piercing understanding.

> I was like a deaf person who could talk; when someone else spoke, I either said nothing or spoke over them on my own track, an express train, stopping at no stations until the end (p. 75).

Yet her problem of incomprehension was not really a problem of inability to comprehend, anymore than Richard's not focusing on the dangers of crossing a road is really a function of not understanding danger, only a difficulty of comprehending at a given moment what other people were comprehending. She was sorting sensory input differently than other people:

> I had no concept for the usefulness of anything but the physical, observable context, such as the room a discussion took place in or whether it was night or day. Who was related to whom, how you came to know them, or what their life story was, was of no use whatsoever to a filing cabinet using its own system (p. 99).

As she worked at consciously thinking about her ways of deriving meaning, she found herself able to comprehend more and more, "seventy percent on a very good day (given a one-to-one conversation, a familiar voice, and familiar surroundings). I began to experience 'self' and 'other' equally at the same time, without fading out, channel switching, or background-foreground effect" (p. 99).

Thus Williams' struggle with understanding is not in her mind a struggle with retardation (i.e. inability to think) but with managing the resources of awareness and thinking. Remarking on the difficulties she has observed in others with autism, including people who have been labeled severely retarded and autistic, Williams cautions that too often,

> those who have trouble linking thought to action or words, or vice versa, are thought retarded or disturbed, when the problem may not be in the capacity so much as the mechanics (pp. 21-22).

She defines her dilemma and that of others with autism as one of systems-management (i.e. integration) and systems-forfeiting. In order to get one thing to work, it is often necessary to abandon or neglect another. For example, the person may have to switch off emotional signals in order to accept factual information, or switch off auditory input to take in visual stimuli.

ON HUMOR AND UNDERSTANDING

Back to Richard and his view of things. His humor reveals a keen awareness of others. As we were out for a drive near a seaside town east of London, we passed a boardwalk.

"I wish I could get my feet up on the table like that," Richard commented.

"You saw somebody relaxed did you?" I asked.

"Yes, it looks very good if you are young enough to get away with it, ha, ha, ha. I dared myself to joke with Doug."

Then Richard added, "I guess I am different from lots of people with autism."

Assuming that he was talking about putting his feet up, I asked, "How so, in terms of having the kind of humor you have?"

But Richard had shifted to a different topic:

"(No) in going forward, forward, forward and never giving up. The children at school gave up trying. They hid inside to stay safe but very frightened to even understand themselves. They look normal but they did not understand their feelings. I saw them hurting but I feared to look like them. No heart, no feelings, no understanding of who they were. Mum told me that I need to keep going no matter what."

In his humor *and* in his reflections on growing up with others with autism, Richard reveals a keen interest in what others are thinking and feeling. He was interested in what I thought of his humor, knowing that people judge each others' humor. He worried about what other children felt, and what could happen when anyone, he especially, decides to give up, rather than to go "forward, forward, forward." Richard's awareness of others' reactions and feelings comes out easily now that he can communicate. Prior to learning to type, it was hard to know his awareness. His facial expressions include a welcoming smile, but he lacks easy modulation of facial features, an important type of communication, and he had no means of sharing complex ideas.

COMPULSIONS AND AWARENESS

Richard struggles with compulsiveness in much the same way that many people with autism do. He has an obsession with electric fans. Whenever he sees a fan he runs toward and inspects it. One day, as we were walking through a mall, he caught sight of a fan in an appliance store and immediately ran toward the store.

There was a young child, perhaps one and a half or two years old, standing in the door watching with some alarm as this young man ran toward her. Later, when Richard's father expressed concern over his having come close to running down the child, Richard remarked:

> I was running to the shop, but I had stopped. Cut my big head off. I understand that she is a baby. I guess I should be more understanding that with children and with older people walking in the garden. Very much effort to break old habits. I guess I should make more effort to break old habits.

I allowed as how it must be hard to always be in control, to which Richard responded, "Okay I guess it is, but I know it is very frightening for the baby to see me dashing towards her like that."

Sean Barron (Barron and Barron, *There's a Boy in Here*, 1992), a person with autism who developed typical speech and who co-authored an autobiographical account of life with autism, reports that repetitive, compulsive acts gave him satisfaction but also kept him from awareness of what others were saying and doing. It wasn't that he could never understand, or that he was incapable of complex thinking. Rather, his compulsive tasks took all his attention:

I remember my mother telling me not to do things I loved, like, "Don't throw your crayons down the register!" I have a very good memory, I think. But what she said had no meaning because what I wanted to do blocked out her words." (P. 21).

As he got older and as his mother and father and others interrupted these compulsions, he was able to shift his attention to other things.

Apparently, Richard Attfield never did tune out completely to the point of giving up on seeking understanding, even though there were many things that confused him about how he experiences the world, especially from a sensory standpoint. In contrast to this, Sue Rubin (1996), a high school student who until the age of 13 was in her words, "tested ... and believed to function at the level of a two year old," had a fuller sense of being preoccupied by her autistic tendencies. She was even in her own mind "really ... retarded." Commenting now on what it was like before she had a way to reach out to the world, Sue Rubin explains her condition as having been one of being consumed by autism. It was when she began to have a way of communicating that her focus and performance changed. She did not change altogether, but she did change in some very significant ways.

> I am very autistic with many awful behaviors including an occasional bout with amazingly life threatening head banging. I speak mostly with echolalia and also am quite antisocial.
> I am assuming an identity of a normal teenager ... Now applying to colleges.

She tempers this announcement with her realization that "wanting to be normal ... Is not enough ... To overcome all the aspects of autism that haunt my days."

Sue Rubin has described the contextual nature of her dual experiences, first with retardation and then with competence:

> It was only after I started typing and my brain somehow started working, that I began to think. Before that I merely reacted to my immediate environment. I must have been absorbing a lot of information because awesome words were at my disposal, but I didn't know what I knew until I was able to type fairly fluently. I also knew some mathematics but was totally ignorant in other areas. Awash in autism and self centeredness I was unable really to connect with people. I am ashamed to say I was totally indifferent to my parents and brother. Although I was aware of their existence they were objects who did things for me. It was not until I started typing that I equated any special significance with my family. Assume also that life was much easier then. I am now aware of the world around me with all of its warts. I constantly worry about all really awful things none of which I can control, like the IRA starting

The Metaphor of Mental Retardation

its bombings again, Hamas in Israel, Buchanan and the radical right who are a danger to people like me who are different. Assume I worry and can't control my emotions so I am always ready to blow up. When I was retarded I sometimes had tantrums but they were over things easier to fix.

Although life is much more challenging now I could never go back to my retarded state.

We who look and act retarded must be freed from our prison.

Sue Rubin's description of her experience contrasts with Richard Attfield's in the sense that he reports being aware of the world even though he too was essentially trapped in silence—Richard was often consumed by his autism, with compulsions, with sensory sensitivities, and with an inability to let people around him know what he was experiencing. But were either Sue or Richard ever retarded? Another way to frame their predicaments would be to say that the contexts in which they found themselves were retarded. In other words, by not understanding what they were experiencing, by not developing scaffolds that would foster their communication, the world and its deficit way of conceptualizing people with autism proved debilitating.

STRUGGLING WITH SENSORY SENSITIVITIES

Richard's struggle to understand his own sensory sensitivities and compulsions is ongoing and, as for any of us who attempt to figure out our reactions to certain events, shifting. One day he tried to explain his fascination with and fear of fans and certain other appliances.

> Okay I guess I get upset if they turned on the fan because I get more terrified of them if they go too fast but that is not it Doug. I would hear the fan, I would get frightened to understand the noise. I would feel terrified. I would hold my breath. And I began to get high from lack of air. That's not right. I had five times the fear after that happened. That gave me a head full of shit.
>
> Yes fear to understand all this. Half understanding. I had fractured sound. I was four and half and I heard noises in my head. That's as near as I can get to describing it. Okay, like a mighty plane taking off. The noise was outside. I thought it was in my head, but I understand. I hope this is right Doug. It was outside of me. I think it was outside, but at the time I thought it was inside. I would just get up and hear it. It seemed to me that... I had fractured sound. I grew up that way. I heard things differently all the time. One day it would sound different to the next. There was no consistency to it. I would get up from the floor, or from the chair and I would hear the noise. That was great noise like a mighty plane. And I would feel like I had to get away from it. But I had no understanding of the fear and so I stayed there and tried to hide

from it. So hug me and tell me it is okay to feel frightened to hear. I was frightened of sounds from that time on. But I grew to understand that it had to be **me,** not the machines. It was not the machines that changed frequency. It was fractured. So one day it was one sound and then it changed to another sound, different to what it had been. I was terrified of the fans, hair dryers, tumble dryers, washing machines, water in pipes at the school. It was not too bad and then it would get worse and worse until I was terrified of the sound of machines at all. And I guess that eventually I understand that it was my hearing and that it was not the machines. And I grew up unable to understand that. But I hear okay now.

Richard's other sensory experiences also left him confused at times:

I would hear a word, understand it, I would get it, I would find the face to it. I would see the object they would tell me to see. I would get it, feel fine, feel certain,, but then it began again, the uncertainty of it. Did they say goodnight or did I hear it differently? This time sounded different to me, not the same as before. I would see different every time. Nothing was safe to understand. Nothing remained consistent. And they thought I was retarded. But I knew I could understand if I was given time to feel, time to see, time to hear.

LIMITING INTAKE TO MAXIMIZE UPTAKE

Some people with autism describe careful listening or attending as an extreme balancing act, keeping certain stimuli at bay while consciously tuning in to another person's spoken words. Williams (1994) reports that she does best in interview conversations if she has seen the other person's questions in writing and if she herself has been able to write out her responses (personal communication). Then she can elaborate from her written words.

Rubin describes the barrage of stimuli that come whenever large groups of people converge as conditions she must escape. "I absolutely dislike being in a crowded room because the noise and activity are overwhelming" (Rubin, 1995, p. B6). Dietmar Zoller (1992), another person who communicates by facilitation describes his similar struggles with sensory overload:

I can't travel downtown by myself. I became aware of this again when I went downtown with my parents yesterday. Most often I let them lead me like a blind man not because I see nothing but because I see too much and then lose my orientation. (Zoller, August 10, 1989).

Even one-to-one relationships can be too much at times, "because the autistic person can't tolerate the other. He always notices too much and becomes over-

whelmed" (Zoller, 1992, Diary entry, June 1989). Zoller explains that the ability to think depends on "structured support" and "on the ability to sort the ever present stimuli" (Diary entry, June, 1989).

Conclusion

THE CONTEXT OF ABILITY: GUIDING PRINCIPLES

Anyone's thinking ability, any measure of intelligence, always occurs in some context. And certain contexts foster optimal performance while others may actually impede performance or make performance impossible. For most of us, the contexts we find ourselves in change frequently, as does our performance (for a discussion of how this has been observed in autism, see Oppenheim, 1974). Over time, we are able to discover the circumstances under which we are most likely to do well. But imagine what it would be like not to know why performance is so difficult or to be unable to communicate to people around you what factors help you do well and which ones set you into a frenzy. Richard Attfield experienced both fates, and so he spent all of his primary and secondary school years being thought of as retarded, even though he was a complex thinker all along. And what happens when a person becomes convinced that he or she cannot be competent, for example cannot achieve a calm state, cannot handle multiple stimuli, cannot attend to the world in the way that other people do, and therefore stops listening to the world's words, as Rubin described above? It wasn't that she was incapable of understanding, only that she wasn't participating in understanding. It wasn't that *she was* retarded, only that she and the world *considered* her so.

We have to wonder for how many the concept and reification of mental retardation masks experiences that are simply misunderstood. While presuming retardation on the part of the other may protect a dominant way of thinking about autism, the presumption of ability is the precondition to hearing how people with autism interpret their own lives. In the words of Larry Bissonnette:

> You cannot learn titling of disability unless you imprint real experiences of people who live with limitations of lasting intensity on property of esteemed scientific inquiry. (Bissonnette, 1997)

And we cannot really know how people experience the world unless they are able to tell us. If we insist on labeling certain behaviors as evidence of mental retardation, even though we cannot in a sure sense *know* what the other person thinks, then we will tend to stop looking for evidence of complex thought. Such labeling is, in Bissonnette's words, "like leasing a car with the destination determined" (Bissonnette, 1997).

Although recent autobiographical accounts by people with autism confirm much of what researchers have previously observed, especially in terms of sensory and motor disturbance issues, most of these accounts make it apparent that the person with autism is not so much retarded as in need of sensitive accommodations. Predictably, this work will be more difficult than providing eyeglasses and/or mobility training to a visually impaired student, hearing aids and/or total communication strategies to a hearing impaired student, a wheelchair to a physically impaired student, or a letter board to a student with cerebral palsy, and may be even more complex and challenging than providing teaching and learning interventions to the student with learning disabilities. The struggle for the field of autism, which must be carried out *with* people with autism, is to continue to find ways of specifying and providing the complex range of accommodations that foster complex thinking and expression.

The following are *Guiding Principles* for creating contexts for communication and participation:

As a matter of basic sensitivity and good educational practice, educators must presume that the person is intelligent. Although the person may be unable to prove this immediately, consistently, or much at all, and may have a severe communication impairment whereby he or she is unable to demonstrate what he or she thinks and feels, or at least has great difficulty in being understood, it is imperative that such individuals not be further handicapped by the attitudes of people whom they encounter. It is especially important that difficulties with demonstrating ability not be taken as evidence of intellectual incompetence.

Related to the presumption of competence, educators have a responsibility to try and find ways to assist the person in bridging the gap between separation from others and participation, between silence or ineffective and even annoying communication and understandable communication, and between inaction or disordered action and meaningful participation.

Presume that the person who has not yet participated in inclusive settings to the extent that his or her non-disabled peers do has a desire to participate fully. Presume that the person desires social interaction even if he or she has difficulty with it.

Presume that the student is paying attention to the people who attempt to interact with him/her, even if signs of this may often seem nonexistent or tenuous.

Presume that students with disabilities, like all other people, may demonstrate abilities in some contexts and not in others. Demonstration of abilities will change across different contexts and over time. The role of the teacher and all others in an educational setting is to understand what contexts help the person participate in rich and complex ways. Within this perspective, competence is not static, but is rather always shifting.

Presume that there are specific things to learn about how someone adapts to specific contexts.

In assessing the effectiveness of participation in academics, it is important to consider not only the student's skills, but also those of the people around him or her, of supportive people in the setting, and the impact of the setting itself, including various environmental features (accessibility, lighting, sound etc.) Professionals who wish to assess inclusion and levels of participation in academics should have extensive background in school inclusion and in academic instruction. And the assessors need to recognize that their role in supporting and interacting with individuals who are expected to participate may strongly influence, either positively or negatively, the outcomes of an assessment; students themselves are often able to collaborate with teachers and others to work out effective strategies for measuring their own progress in academics.

Presume that students already have within themselves many of the experiences, skills, and knowledge that enable them to be active learners in a context that values dialogue. This perspective recognizes that students can be leaders in their own education.

References

Baldac, S., and Parsons, C. (1995). Factors affecting performance in facilitated communication. In Biklen, D., & Cardinal, D., (Eds.), *Contested words, contested science.* New York, Teachers College Press, 79-95.

Baron-Cohen, S. (1996) *Mindblindness: An essay on autism and theory of mind.* Cambridge, MA: MIT Press.

Barron, J. & Barron, S. (1992). *There's a boy in here.* New York: Simon & Schuster.

Biklen, D. (1993) *Communication unbound.* New York: Teachers College Press.

Biklen, D. & Cardinal, D.N (Eds.) (1997). *Contested words, contested science: Unraveling the facilitated communication controversy.* New York: Teachers College Press.

Bissonnette, L. (1996) Submission to the Administration on Developmental Disabilities/Office of Special Education and Rehabilitation Services Panel on Facilitated Communication.

Bissonnette, L. (1997) Maine Conference on Facilitation. Portland: University of Maine U.A.P.

Cardinal, D., Hanson, D., & Wakeham, J. (1996). An investigation of authorship in facilitated communication. *Mental Retardation,* 34 (4), 231-242.

Crossley, R. (1994). *Facilitated communication training.* New York: Teachers College Press.

Crossley, R. & McDonald, A. (1980). *Annie's coming out.* New York: Penguin.

Crossley, R. & Remington-Gumey, J. (1992). Getting the words out: Facilitated communication training. *Topics in Language Disorders,* 12 (4), 29-45.

Dwyer, J. (1996). Access to justice for people with severe communication impairment. *Australian Journal of Administrative Law,* 3 (2), 73-120.

Eastham, M. (1992). *Silent words.* Ottawa: Oliver Pate.

Eberlin, M., McConnachie, G., Ibel, S., & Volpe, L. (1993). Facilitated communication: A failure to replicate the phenomenon. *Journal of Autism and Developmental Disorders,* 23, (3), 507-530.

Grandin, T. & Scariano, M.N. (1986). *Emergence labeled autistic.* Novato, CA: Arena Press.

Jacobson, J. W., Mulick, J.A., and Schwartz, A.A. (1995). A history of facilitated communication: Science, pseudoscience, and antiscience, *American Psychologist,* 50 (9), 750-765.

Kangas, K.A. & Lloyd, L.L. (1988). Early cognitive skills as prerequisites to augmentative and alternative communication use: What are we waiting for? *Augmentative and Alternative Communication,* 4, 211-221.

Klewe, L. (I 993). Brief report: An empirical evaluation of spelling boards as a means of communication for the multihandicapped. *Journal of Developmental Disorders,* 23 (3), 559-566.

Lane, H. (1980). *Helen and teacher.* New York: Delacorte Press/Seymour Lawrence.

Marcus, E. & Shevin, M. (I 997). Sorting it out under fire: Our journey. In D. Biklen and D.N. Cardinal (Eds.) *Contested words, contested science.* New York: Teachers College Press, 115-134.

Nolan, C. (1987). *Under the eve of the clock.* New York: St. Martins Press.

Olney, M. (1995). *A controlled evaluation of facilitated communication.* Unpublished doctoral dissertation, Syracuse University, Syracuse, New York.

Oppenheim, R. (1974). *Effective teaching methods for autistic children.* Springfield, IL: Thomas.

Rapin, L. (1997). Current concepts: Autism. *The New England Journal of Medicine.* 337 (2), 97-104.

Regal, R.A., Rooney, J.R., & Wandas, T. (I 994). Facilitated communication: An experimental evaluation. *Journal of Autism and Developmental Disorders* 24 (3), 345-355.

Rubin, S. (June 12, 1995a). *Battling for the disabled with Cesar Chavez in Mind, Los Angeles Times,* B6.

Rubin, S. (1995b). *On doing one's homework.... Facilitated communication digest,* 4 (1), 1..

Rubin, S. (1996) Submission to the Administration on Developmental Disabilities/Office of Special Education and Rehabilitation Services Panel on Facilitated Communication.

Sheehan, C. & Matuozzi, R. (1996). Validation of facilitated communication. *Mental Retardation,* 34(2), 94-107.

Sienkiewicz-Mercer, R. & Kaplan, S. B. (1989). *I raise my eyes to say yes.* Boston: Houghton Mifflin.

Smith, M.D., & Belcher, R.G. (1993). Facilitated communication: The effects of facilitator knowledge and level of assistance on output. *Journal of Autism and Developmental Disorders,* 24 (3), 357-367.

Weiss, M.i. S., Wagner, S., & Bauman, M. (I 996). A case of validated facilitated communication. *Mental Retardation,* 34 (4), 220-230.

Wheeler, D.L., Jacobson, J.W., Paglieri, R.A., & Schwartz, A.A. (1993). An experimental assessment of facilitated communication. *Mental Retardation,* 31 (1), 49-60.

Williams, D. (1994). *Somebody somewhere.* New York: Times Mirror.

Zeigler, A.L., Thierry, D., & Calame, A. (1990). Hidden intelligence of multiply handicapped child with Joubert syndrome. *Developmental Medicine and Child Neurology,*3-2, 261-266.

Zoller, Dietmar (I 992). *Ich gebe nichtauf (I won't give up).* Bem: Scherz Verlag. (Translations by Annegret Schubert)

SECTION II

Legal Issues

5

From Deficiency to Equality

How are Canada's New Constitutional Protections Working for Persons with Disabilities?

Orville Endicott
York University, Toronto, Ontario

No one can predict as a human being is born where the limits of that person's growth and development will be.... What we call the inability of persons with severe handicaps to communicate may well be our ineptness in listening.
From Gunnar Dybwad's response upon receiving an honorary degree of Doctor of Human Letters from Temple University, February 12, 1977

Introduction

The words quoted above reflect realities which have been proclaimed very effectively over the years by the pioneer advocate who spoke them more than two decades ago. Their simple essence is that we have no business jumping to conclusions about some people's inferiority to others. They are words which are gradually sinking into our collective consciousness. This chapter is about one country's experience in attempting to translate the essential meaning of those ideas into the wording of its fundamental laws.

In 1982 the *Canadian Charter of Rights and Freedoms* became part of Canada's Constitution.[1] Section 15(1) of the *Charter* reads as follows:

> Every individual is equal before and under the law and has the right to the equal protection and equal benefit of the law without discrimination and, in particular, without discrimination based on race, national or ethnic origin, colour, religion, sex, age or *mental or physical disability*.[2] (emphasis added)

With the enactment of the *Charter*, Canada became the first country in the world to include in its constitution a specific guarantee of legal equality for persons with disabilities.[3]

It was not until more than ten years later that litigation based on the constitutional equality protections for persons with disabilities began to reach the Supreme Court of Canada. Two cases involving questions of discrimination by agents of government on grounds of disability have now been decided. In 1996 the Court heard an appeal from a decision of the Court of Appeal for Ontario in the case of *Eaton v. Brant County Board of Education*,[4] in which the parents of a young girl with both physical and intellectual disabilities argued that she had a constitutional right to be educated, with appropriate supports, in the same classroom in her neighbourhood school with other, non-disabled children. In 1997 a decision was handed down in *Eldridge et al. v. Attorney General of British Columbia*,[5] in which a group of deaf persons complained that they were wrongly denied the services of a sign-language interpreter when they sought the care of a physician under that Province's universal health insurance plan.[6]

The respective outcomes of these two cases are challenging to reconcile. Emily Eaton and her parents were told that being required to be educated in a segregated special class for children with disabilities, on the facts of Emily's case, is not discriminatory under the *Charter*. Susan Eldridge and her friends were granted the right to have an interpreter, provided at government expense, in any situation in which a hearing patient would expect to enjoy full and free communication with his or her health care practitioner. Notwithstanding their seemingly opposite outcomes, the judicial opinions in both of these cases offer a great deal of material to enlarge our understanding of what the constitutional guarantee of equality in Canada will ultimately mean.

The greater part of this chapter is a critical examination of the Supreme Court of Canada's decision in the *Eaton* case. The *Eldridge* decision is discussed more briefly as an indicator of some positive development in the Court's thinking about constitutional equality in the year following the release of the *Eaton* judgment.

Eaton v. Brant County Board of Education

History of the Litigation

This case originated in the early 1990's when Emily Eaton's parents were unsuccessful in persuading the Brant County (Ontario) Board of Education that she should attend a regular class in her neighbourhood school. The Board determined that her disabilities, related to cerebral palsy, were such that it was in her best interests to be placed in a special class for children with disabilities in another public school in the area. The Eatons pursued the matter through the administrative appeal process set out in a Regulation under the Ontario *Education Act*.[7] At every level their request that Emily be included with typical children in a regular class was refused.

A Special Education Tribunal ruled against the parents in November, 1993. It was argued before the Tribunal on behalf of the Eatons that inclusion in a regular class was Emily's right by virtue of the equality guarantee in s. 15(1) of the *Canadian Charter of Rights and Freedoms*.[8]

Before the dispute was heard by the Special Education Tribunal, the Eatons obtained an injunction from the Ontario Court (General Division) requiring the School Board to keep Emily in the regular classroom until the decision of the Tribunal was known. This meant that she spent the first three years of her schooling in the same classroom with her non-disabled peers, in a school operated by her adversaries in the litigation, the Brant County Board of Education. Upon receiving the judgment of the Tribunal endorsing the School Board's decision to place Emily in a segregated special class in another school, her parents moved her to a school operated by the Brant County Roman Catholic Separate School Board, where she continues, five years later, to attend a regular class.

An application by the Eatons for Judicial Review of the Special Education Tribunal decision was dismissed by the Divisional Court of the Ontario Court of Justice. Leave to appeal to the Court of Appeal for Ontario was obtained, and on February 15, 1995, the Court of Appeal handed down its unanimous judgment, allowing the appeal on the grounds that

> the *Charter* requires that, regardless of its perceived pedagogical merit, a non-consensual exclusionary placement be recognized as discriminatory and not be resorted to unless alternatives are proven inadequate.[9]

The Court of Appeal for Ontario was satisfied that, if inclusive education is "reasonably capable of meeting the child's special needs",[10] then the constitutional equality guarantee should mean that the child has the right to be placed in a regular class.

The Appeal Court, acting on its own motion, placed the blame for the constitutional violation on the province's *legislation*, which provides for (but does not require) children to be excluded from the regular classroom, contrary to their equality rights. Emily Eaton's parents had argued that it was the decision of the School Board's representatives and of the Special Education Tribunal which constituted the discrimination, rather than any flaw in the legislation itself.

The Brant County Board of Education then obtained leave to appeal the decision of the provincial Court of Appeal to the Supreme Court of Canada. The appeal to the Supreme Court was joined by twelve intervener groups (*amici curiae*), including several provincial ministries of education and nine children's and disability rights advocacy groups. The appeal was heard on October 8, 1996. The central issue before the Supreme Court was whether Emily Eaton's exclusion from a regular class contravened her equality rights under the *Canadian Charter of Rights and Freedoms*.

The day following the hearing, the Supreme Court unanimously allowed the School Board's appeal, effectively ruling that requiring Emily Eaton to attend a special class for pupils with disabilities did not violate her constitutional right to equality under section 15(1) of the *Charter*. The Court's ruling was accompanied by an announcement that reasons for the decision would follow. On February 6, 1997, those reasons were released.

Reasons for Judgment

The Supreme Court allowed the School Board's appeal in the *Eaton* case on three separate grounds, one procedural, another a matter of statutory interpretation, and the other substantive. The substantive ground was the finding that Emily Eaton had not been discriminated against in violation of her constitutional right to equality. Both the procedural ground and that involving a principle of statutory interpretation can be traced to the insistence of the Court of Appeal for Ontario, once it found that Emily *had* been discriminated against, that the blame for the *Charter* violation should be attributed to the legislation, rather than to the decision of the School Board and the Special Education Tribunal that she should be placed in a segregated setting. These issues were unfortunate red herrings that had nothing to do with whether forced school segregation is in fact discriminatory.

The question of primary interest in the *Eaton* case is in what circumstances exclusion of a child with a disability from the regular classroom is a denial of his or her equality rights as stated in the *Canadian Charter of Rights and Freedoms*. It is important to bear in mind that the Court might have come to a different conclusion in Emily Eaton's case if the factual record had provided any insight into her positive experiences of inclusion in the regular Separate School classroom which she had attended since the Special Education Tribunal handed down its decision three years earlier. The only evidence before the Court, apart from that of her parents, pertaining to her experience in an integrated classroom, came from witnesses who were employees of the appellant School Board that had been forced to keep her there by the lower Court's injunction.

I. THE ISSUE OF BEST INTERESTS AS A TEST OF EQUALITY

In the *Eaton* case, the Special Education Tribunal defined its task as being to determine "whether Emily Eaton's special needs can be met best in a regular class or in a special class".[11] This theory of the case seems to have been based on the assumption that Emily's right to equality and her right to receive the best possible education can be treated as one and the same. Although the Tribunal concluded that her educational needs could only be met effectively in a segregated class, there was very little evidence to support that contention. The Supreme Court admitted as much in its reasons for judgment.[12]

For close to a decade, the Supreme Court's test of whether a law or government action is discriminatory within the meaning of section 15(1) of the *Charter* has been to ask whether a distinction has been made on the basis of a prohibited ground (in this case disability) that has the effect of withholding a benefit from the person that would not be withheld from other persons, or of imposing a burden or disadvantage on the person that would not be imposed on other persons. If these adverse effects are not experienced, then the distinction that was made does not constitute discrimination, and the *Charter* guarantee of equality has not been violated.[13] Thus, the central issue in the *Eaton* case was whether placing Emily in a segregated special class would amount to the withholding of a benefit enjoyed by other pupils in a regular class, or the imposition of a burden to which typical students are not subjected, or both. Defining the issue in this manner begs the question of whether "benefit" is to be assessed in terms of academic achievement alone, or also in terms of achieving equality in a broader social sense. The Supreme Court chose to keep the focus very narrow.

Madam Justice Arbour, writing for the Court of Appeal for Ontario in *Eaton*, adopted a broad approach to the notions of benefit and disadvantage. She took into account the larger "social, historical and political context" which revealed "that the history of disabled persons, which the *Charter* seeks to redress and prevent, is a history of exclusion".[14] It was her opinion that equality is a principle that operates on a higher level than educational best interests. The latter are based on pragmatic considerations of what educational practices are most likely to generate the best learning outcomes for the individual pupil. Equality, it can be argued, is an over-arching concept that includes best interests, but extends much further than the immediate context of the service being offered. In education, it is the principle that requires that everything be done by the school to ensure that children with disabilities are regarded and treated as equals with all other children, and that they will continue to enjoy that equality beyond their school years.

Justice Sopinka concluded that "Integration can be either a benefit or a burden depending on whether the individual can profit from the advantages that integration provides".[15] This "either/or" analysis obscures the complexity of the notion of benefits and burdens. In reality, the weighing of the benefits and burdens of inclusive education (as is the case with many other equality issues) is a multi-facetted exercise, in which the *net* benefit or *net* disadvantage should be the determinative factor. While there may have been offsetting burdens faced by Emily Eaton in the regular class, what was actually done to minimize those burdens and to permit the balance to be tipped in favour of the inherent benefits of inclusion? This is the nexus between best interests and reasonable accommodation, which will be addressed below.

Justice Arbour believed that the inherent benefits of true inclusion will always outweigh any burdens that may accompany integration for a particular child:

> School officials cannot simply apply a test of "best interest of the child". Such a test could prove insensitive to the equality rights of the child, which, when

asserted, may trump what would otherwise appear to others to be in the child's best interest.[16]

In his analysis of the substantive issue of discrimination, Justice Sopinka addressed his mind to the same historical context that had so influenced Justice Arbour's judgment in the Court of Appeal. Justice Sopinka stated,

> A change of attitude with respect to disabled persons was initiated by the report of Walter B. Williston entitled *Present Arrangements for the Care and Supervision of Mentally Retarded Persons in Ontario* (1971). With it came a recognition of the desirability of integration and de-institutionalization. The change in attitude was reflected in the *Education Act*.[17]

What Justice Sopinka failed to do was to consider this historical reality as part of the current equation in calculating benefits and burdens for Emily Eaton. He evidently assumed that the "change of attitude" he referred to as having been "initiated" a quarter of a century earlier, had in fact been *complete* by the time the Eatons began their dispute with the Brant County School Board. This is manifestly not the case. The question of attitudes leads into the next major theme in the Supreme Court's reasons for judgment.

II. STEREOTYPES AND IRRELEVANCIES

Justice Sopinka noted that in previous equality rights decisions,[18] the Supreme Court had subscribed to the principle that, when an individual is treated on the basis of stereotypes, rather than the actual characteristics of the person, then inequality will result because the stereotypical characteristics are by definition *irrelevant* as a basis on which to make distinctions. Some Supreme Court Justices seemed to go so far as to say that without stereotypes there is no discrimination. However, in the *Andrews* case cited above,[19] the Supreme Court said that the test for discrimination under s. 15 of the *Charter* was whether the complainant experienced adverse effects as a consequence of a distinction made between him and persons who do not share his protected characteristic (in that case foreign citizenship as a barrier to practising law in a Canadian province). As in earlier non-*Charter* discrimination cases,[20] the intent or the stereotypical thinking of the person responsible for the discrimination was of no consequence. A finding of discrimination was based on the adverse impact on the complainant, not on the mental processes of the person alleged to have been responsible for the discrimination.

In *Eaton*, the Supreme Court appears to have been heavily influenced by its view that Emily Eaton's disability *was* relevant to the distinction made by the School Board in consigning her to a separate class. The relevance principle was summed up by Justice Sopinka: "In general, distinctions based on presumed rather than actual characteristics are the hallmarks of discrimination". He went on to say that this principle has "particular significance when applied to physical and mental disability".[21] Disability frequently requires differential treatment in order to *protect* the equality rights of the individual. As opposed to treating people differently because of characteristics they do not really possess (i.e. stereotypes), where disability is involved, people may have to be treated differently because they really *are* different, and their actual differences from other people are *relevant* to decisions about how they should be treated. It is the nature of such differences that dictates the kind of accommodations they require in order to obtain equal benefit from a publicly funded service, such as education. Justice Sopinka referred to this issue as "the 'difference dilemma'" by which he appears to have meant that the same treatment may violate the equality rights of one person with a disability, but protect the equality rights of another.

The Supreme Court of Canada in *Eaton* discounted the fact that persons with disabilities can become victims of discrimination *both* because their real characteristics are not properly accommodated, *and* because they are dealt with in terms of stereotypes that do not correspond to the realities of their lives. Justice Sopinka does say that "in the case of disability . . . one of the objectives (is) the elimination of discrimination by the attribution of untrue characteristics based on stereotypical attitudes".[22] Indeed, he appeared to give this approach equal billing with that which says that real differences in the lives of people with disabilities must be accommodated. However, before ending this paragraph in his judgment, he wrote, "The discrimination inquiry which uses 'the attribution of stereotypical characteristics' reasoning as commonly understood *is simply inappropriate here*".[23] It is hard to avoid the conclusion that Justice Sopinka has first asserted and then denied the relevance of stereotypical attitudes to the determination of the existence of discrimination on the ground of mental disability.

According to Justice Sopinka, the "true characteristics of this group . . . act as *headwinds* to the enjoyment of society's benefits".[24] The imagery of "headwinds" that impede the progress of a person with disabilities is interesting, and even insightful, so long as these headwinds are not viewed as originating solely, or even primarily, from the individual's personal impairments. Headwinds, in actuality and by definition, originate outside of persons and are directed against them as a result of atmospheric (read "environmental") conditions. To identify the headwinds with the "true characteristics of this group" (i.e. persons with disabilities) does violence to an otherwise useful metaphor. The *prevailing* headwinds that have held people with disabilities back in our society are those emanating from the negative attitudes and practices of those individuals and agencies in society that disempower, segregate and marginalise them, rather than accepting people with disabilities and identifying the special measures required in order to help them fulfil their ordinary needs and meet their personal potential. Justice Sopinka in fact articulated this reality very well in the sentence that follows the introduction of his "headwinds" analogy:

> Exclusion from the mainstream of society results from the construction of a society based solely on "mainstream" attributes to which disabled persons will never be able to gain access.[25]

Surely it is "the construction of a society" such as he described that gives rise to the "headwinds".

In the following paragraph, Justice Sopinka revisited the historical "evolution of special education in Ontario". He wrote,

> The earlier policy of exclusion ... was influenced in large part by a stereotypical attitude to disabled persons.... No account was taken of the true characteristics of individual members of the disabled population, nor was any attempt made to accommodate these characteristics.[26]

He then credited once again the 1971 Williston Report "and other developments" as having produced a "change of attitude", as a result of which educational policy in Ontario shifted from one based on stereotypes to one based on the need for accommodation. Justice Sopinka seems to have believed that this change of attitude was complete – a *sea* change, a paradigm shift that corrected all the inequalities that had existed until then. If stereotypical attitudes towards persons with disabilities could produce discrimination as recently as two or three decades earlier, why, we must ask, could they be ruled out in 1997?

There is no question that disability, and particularly intellectual disability, is «relevant» to decisions about how a child should be educated. What the Eatons vainly hoped the Supreme Court would understand is that her disability is *not* relevant to *where* a child like Emily should be educated. The assumption that disability requires segregated placement is, to the Eatons and their supporters, evidence in itself of stereotypical thinking, and thus at the very heart of discrimination.

III. REASONABLE ACCOMMODATION

Having laid to rest any notion that negative attitudes or stereotyping could possibly have been at work in the treatment accorded Emily Eaton by the Brant County Board of Education and the Special Education Tribunal, Justice Sopinka turned his attention to the only other heading under which inequality could be found – the failure to accommodate her particular educational needs. The equality principle of reasonable accommodation has been referred to earlier because it is inextricably linked to both the principles of best interests and of avoiding treating people on the basis of stereotypes.

As noted above, Justice Sopinka believed that reasonable accommodation had become the rule once the Ontario *Education Act* was amended in the 1980's. He summarized those amendments as meaning that

> Integration was the preferred accommodation but if the pupil could not benefit from integration a special program was designed to enable disabled pupils to receive the benefits of education which were available to others.[27]

Here, as elsewhere in his judgment, Justice Sopinka seems to equate "special" education with "segregated" education. Regardless of their position with respect to the value of inclusion of pupils with disabilities in regular classes, all educators recognize that "special education" is used to describe modifications in the teaching of exceptional pupils in *whatever* setting it takes place. Many educators now take the position that the education of children with disabilities should not be called "special education", largely because it denotes a mind-set that emphasizes differences both among pupils and among instructional strategies and methods, not to mention a bias in favour of segregated placement. The confusion in Justice Sopinka's judgment between "special education" and "segregated education" is more than a mere misunderstanding of the terminology. It betrays a very limited grasp on the part of the Supreme Court of the potential application of the principle of accommodation in this area.

Reference has been made above to the strong relationship between the best interests (benefits-versus-burdens) principle of equality jurisprudence and the reasonable accommodation principle. It is impossible to say that a particular approach is not in an individual's "best interests" without having first determined whether the agency responsible has exerted its *best efforts* to accommodate that individual's personal needs.

It is important to note that the Court endorsed the principle which Justice Sopinka (wrongly) thought was incorporated in current law and policy in Ontario, as noted above, that "integration (is) the preferred accommodation".[28] On behalf of the Court, Justice Sopinka wrote, "*Integration should be recognized as the norm of general application because of the benefits it generally provides*".[29] Unfortunately, the foregoing statement is just the first clause of a single sentence in Justice Sopinka's judgment. The sentence concludes, "a presumption in favour of integrated schooling would work to the disadvantage of pupils who require special education in order to achieve equality". Once again, it is clear that the Supreme Court mistakenly regarded "special" education as meaning "segregated" education. It is as though integration, while it may be the "preferred accommodation", stands by itself and does not admit other forms of accommodation within the context of the integrated classroom. The Eatons were clearly not claiming that Emily has a constitutional right to be placed in a regular classroom without any additional supports or accommodations to her exceptional learning needs.

No one could possibly believe that a child with any significant cognitive impairment can benefit from regular class placement *by itself*. In fact, integration should not be called "accommodation" at all, in that it simply provides the *situation* in which more and more parents and educators believe the child's special learning needs can best be accommodated. The Supreme Court's view of integration was a distorted one, as revealed by Justice Sopinka's belief that the regular classroom is a kind of Procrustean bed that will not fit the dimensions of some children's needs.

IV. THE ROLE OF PARENTS IN PLACEMENT DECISIONS

As one of his reasons for rejecting the Ontario Appeal Court's finding that there is a presumption in favour of inclusion in a regular class as the equality right of every child, Justice Sopinka listed the problems that might arise if parents were given the authority (which the Court of Appeal effectively gave them) to decide whether their child will actually exercise that right. He wrote,

> I would ... question the view that a presumption as to the best interests of a child is a constitutional imperative when the presumption can be automatically displaced by the decision of the child's parents. Such a result runs counter to decisions of this Court that the parents' view of their child's best interests is not dispositive of the question.[30]

One of the cases cited is *E. (Mrs.) v Eve*,[31] in which the Supreme Court unanimously ruled that a mother could not be given the authority to consent to a non-therapeutic sterilization procedure for her daughter, who had an intellectual disability.

For the Supreme Court in *Eaton*, it was more important to try to determine "the appropriate accommodation for an exceptional child ... from a subjective, child-centred perspective, one which attempts to make equality meaningful from the child's point of view as opposed to that of the adults in his or her life."[32] The Court did not address the question of who is in the best position to interpret the actual wishes of a child like Emily Eaton. Ordinarily this is surely the parents.

Parents who take the equality rights of their child seriously enough to engage in litigation to protect those rights, can reasonably be regarded as having a primary concern to see that their child's personal views and preferences, however expressed, are given as much respect and weight as possible in decision making. This is the very *raison d'etre* of equality seeking. In the *Eve* case, the Supreme Court (although it was not a case based on *Charter* equality protections) essentially found against the mother because her wish to impose sterilization on her daughter was a *derogation* of the daughter's equality rights. The effect of the *Eve* decision is that the right to consent or to withhold consent to a non-therapeutic sterilization belongs equally and personally to every individual.

Even for the Court of Appeal, the opinions of the parents were not the final word on whether or not the exclusion of Emily Eaton from the regular class amounted to discrimination contrary to s. 15 of the *Charter*. The parents were entitled to *assert* Emily's rights, but ultimately it was for the courts to determine just *what* those rights are. As Justice Arbour wrote,

Although one should not ignore the intended recipient's perception of whether the measure designed to enhance her equality is in fact a burden rather than a benefit, that subjective perception is not in itself determinative of the issue.[33]

In other words, the test of equality remains that of whether the person has been objectively disadvantaged (i.e. had her best interests compromised) by the differential treatment.

CONCLUSIONS REGARDING *EATON*

The Brant County Board of Education won its appeal to the Supreme Court of Canada because the Court believed that placing Emily Eaton in a special segregated class would produce the best educational outcome for her. The Eatons failed to satisfy the *Andrews*[34] test that, in order to show that you have been discriminated against contrary to s. 15(1) of the *Charter*, you have to prove that you have had a burden imposed on you or a benefit denied you on the basis of your protected characteristic, in this case disability. In reaching its conclusion, the Court adopted a narrow concept of the benefits of public education for a child with a disability. Virtually no account was taken of the burdens associated with exclusion and segregation. The role of parents as interpreters of what their non-verbal children's wishes are with respect to inclusion was minimized.

In addition, the Court viewed the actions of the School Board as being motivated only by Emily's actual limitations, and not in any way by imagined or stereotypical perceptions of how she might best be educated. Having made what the Court regarded as a realistic assessment of Emily's needs, the Court accepted the School Board's position that they could not accommodate those needs in a regular class. Consequently, even though there was virtually no evidence as to how her needs would be accommodated in a segregated setting, the Court concluded that integration was the least preferred form of accommodation. No consideration was given to the question of whether inclusion was working out well for her in the regular Separate School class she has now attended for five years.

The Court also failed to give adequate consideration to the social facts regarding the status of persons with intellectual disabilities in general. While the Court recognized that such persons have been victimized in the past because of negative attitudes and stereotypes, the fact that these attitudes continue to affect their treatment in the 1990's was essentially dismissed.

Eldridge v. Attorney General of British Columbia[35]

The most obvious distinction that can be made between the *Eaton* and the *Eldridge* cases is that Emily Eaton's parents complained that her equality rights were violated because she was being treated by the Brant County Board of Education *differently* from other pupils who did not have significant disabilities, whereas Susan Eldridge's complaint was that she was being treated in the *same manner* as hearing patients by being denied the services of an interpreter, and consequently was receiving a lesser benefit from British Columbia's publicly funded health care system.

A second and related difference between the two cases was that in Emily Eaton's case there was legislation that expressly provided for distinctions to be made on the basis of a child's disability. In *Eldridge* the legislation made no such distinction. Notwithstanding this difference between the legislative provisions involved in the two cases, the principal focus in each case was not on the validity of the legislation, but on the manner in which public officials exercised the discretion they were given under their respective statutes. The Supreme Court has now made it quite clear that legislation that is capable of being read in a manner that permits compliance with *Charter* guarantees is not invalid.

Another important distinction between the two cases is that *Eldridge* involved equality protection based on *physical* disability, whereas *Eaton* was primarily regarded as a *mental* disability case. It is inherently more difficult for judges to imagine what it is like to have a mental disability than to have a physical disability.

Justice La Forest made only two references to the *Eaton* decision in his reasons for judgment in *Eldridge*. Both decisions acknowledged the long-standing position of the Supreme Court that no one can complain of unequal treatment unless the treatment they complain of disadvantages them relative to other persons. Clearly, having the assistance of an interpreter would be in a deaf person's best interests when consulting a physician. Such services would intuitively protect against misdiagnosis and ineffective treatment. Where *Eldridge* parted company from *Eaton* was on the issue of whether the complainants' disabilities were *relevant* to the differential services to which they were subjected. In *Eldridge*, Justice La Forest was able to say, "There is no question that the distinction here is based on a personal characteristic that is irrelevant to the functional values underlying the health care system."[36] In other words, being deaf did not naturally *require* Susan Eldridge to be treated by medical practitioners who lacked full communication with her. In *Eaton*, on the other hand, the Supreme Court concluded that having the type and degree of disabilities Emily Eaton had was fully relevant to the question of whether she should be placed in a segregated special class.

In both *Eaton* and *Eldridge* the Court commented on the social and historical context in which persons with disabilities have endured systemic discrimination. As has been pointed out, those comments seemed to have little impact on the decision that a segregated school placement for Emily Eaton was not a perpetuation of that larger social and historical discrimination, even though years of exclusion from the company of one's non-disabled peers in school presumably does more to perpetuate the systemic problem than would the occasional private consultation between a deaf person and her family doctor without the assistance of an interpreter, however risky that might be for the patient at that particular time.

However that may be, Justice La Forest revisited the historical context of disability and inequality as calling for a broad remedial measure on the part of the Court:

> It is an unfortunate truth that the history of disabled persons in Canada is largely one of exclusion and marginalization. Persons with disabilities have too often been excluded from the labour force, denied access to opportunities for social interaction and advancement, subjected to invidious stereotyping and relegated to institutions.... This historical disadvantage has to a great extent been shaped and perpetuated by the notion that disability is an abnormality or flaw. As a result, disabled persons have not generally been afforded the "equal concern, respect and consideration" that s. 15(1) of the *Charter* demands. Instead, they have been subjected to paternalistic attitudes of pity and charity, and their entrance into the social mainstream has been conditional upon their emulation of able-bodied norms.... One consequence of these attitudes is the persistent social and economic disadvantage faced by the disabled. Statistics indicate that persons with disabilities, in comparison to non-disabled persons, have less education, are more likely to be outside the labour force, face much higher unemployment rates, and are concentrated at the lower end of the pay scale when employed.[37]

A great deal of the foregoing paragraph seems to apply as much to Emily Eaton's situation as it does to Susan Eldridge's. What clearly remains for advocates of inclusive education for children with intellectual disabilities is to make the connections between segregation and inclusion and the "unfortunate truth" that Justice La Forest so eloquently recited.

Notes

1. *The Canadian Charter of Rights and Freedoms*, Part I, *Constitution Act 1982*, Schedule B, *Canada Act 1982*, 1982, c. 11 (U.K.).
2. *Charter*, s. 15(1).
3. The only other countries to have done so, to the best of the author's knowledge, are Germany, which amended Article 3(3) of its Basic Law (the constitutional equality provision) in 1996 to include the words "No one may be disadvantaged because of his disability", and South Africa, where section 9(3) of the Constitution that came into effect on February 7, 1997 reads, in part, "The state may not unfairly discriminate directly or indirectly against anyone on one or more grounds, including ... disability".
4. *Eaton v. Brant County Board of Education*, [1997] 1 S.C.R. 241.
5. *Eldridge v. British Columbia (Attorney General)*, [1997] 3 S.C.R. 624.
6. *Hospital Insurance Act*, R.S.B.C. 1996, c. 204, and *Medical Protection Act*, R.S.B.C. 1996, c. 286.
7. *Education Act*, R.S.O. 1990, c. E-2, ss. 1, 8(3) and R.R.O. 1990, Reg. 305, s. 6(1), (2).
8. Note 2 above.
9. *Eaton v. Brant County Board of Education* (1995), 22 O.R. (3d) 1, at 22a (Court of Appeal).
10. *Ibid.*, p. 21b.

11   The decision of the Special Education Tribunal is not reported.
12   *Eaton* (Supreme Court), Note 4 above, paras. 73, 75.
13   *Andrews v. Law Society of British Columbia*, [1989] 1 S.C.R. 143.
14   *Eaton* (Court of Appeal), Note 9 above, p. 13g,h.
15   *Eaton* (Supreme Court), Note 4 above, para. 69.
16   *Eaton* (Court of Appeal), Note 9 above, p. 10c.
17   *Eaton* (Supreme Court), Note 4 above, para. 58.
18   *Miron v. Trudel*, [1995] 2 S.C.R. 513, and *Egan v. Canada*, [1995] 2 S.C.R. 513.
19   Note 13.
20   *Re Ontario Human Rights Commission and Simpsons-Sears*, [1985] 2 S.C.R. 536, and *Bhinder v. Canadian National Railway Co.*, [1985] 2 S.C.R. 561).
21   *Eaton* (Supreme Court), Note 4 above, para. 66.
22   *Ibid.*, para. 67.
23   *Ibid.*, emphasis added.
24   *Ibid.*, emphasis added.
25   *Ibid.*, para. 67.
26   *Ibid.*, para. 68.
27   *Ibid.*, para. 68.
28   It was not until September 1, 1998 that the Ontario government promulgated a new Regulation for the "Identification and Placement of Exceptional Pupils" that stipulates that, if "placement in a regular class, with appropriate special education services, would meet the pupil's needs, and is consistent with parental preferences ... the committee *shall* decide in favour of placement in a regular class" (Ontario Regulation 181/98, s. 17, emphasis added).
29   *Eaton* (Supreme Court), Note 4 above, para. 68, emphasis added.
30   *Ibid.*, para. 79.
31   [1986] 2 S.C.R. 388.
32   *Eaton*, (Supreme Court), Note 5 above, para. 77.
33   *Eaton* (Court of Appeal), Note 10 above, p. 13f.
34   Note 13.
35   Note 5 above.
36   *Ibid.*, para. 59.
37   *Eldridge* (Supreme Court), Note 5 above, para. 56.

6

The Rights Revolution
From Isolation To Wyatt, Wyoming, And Beyond

Stanley S. Herr
University of Maryland Law School, Baltimore, MD

Introduction

This chapter recounts the rights revolution Gunnar Dybwad helped to inspire. It offers an overview of the legal rights campaign — now over a quarter century old — to curb institutional abuses and support community living. Part I presents the grotesque history that prompted a human rights movement to aid some of society's most vulnerable citizens. Part II then turns to the ethical foundations of this movement. Part III discusses the first modern precedent involving the right to counsel for a person with mental retardation. Part IV explores the core legal milestones: significance of *Wyatt v. Stickney* (1972) and the line of mental retardation institution cases that followed, as well as the significance *of Mills v. Board of Education* (1972), the pioneering right to education case. To demonstrate how far the recognition of such rights has spread, Part V then reviews the alternative dispute resolution model for change used in a federal class action captioned *Weston v. Wyoming State Training School* (1994). Part VI then identifies some of the attributes of a rural state that can mitigate the double jeopardy of age and developmental disabilities, stressing that both the aging and disability services networks must cooperate to serve those who seek the promise of community living. Part VII concludes by observing

---

Acknowledgments: This chapter is in tribute to the splendid mentorship I have received from Rosemary and Gunnar Dybwad. Part of this chapter is a completely revised version of a speech first presented to and printed by the Wyoming Institute for Disabilities/UAP. The names of clients identified only by first names are pseudonyms to protect their confidentiality. For their editing assistance, the author gratefully acknowledges Keith A. Miller, Ph.D., Professor of Social Work and Executive Director of WIND, Sister Kathryn Jennings of Noah House, Pamela DiPesa of the University of Maryland School of Social Work, and Colleen Hogan and Josh Udler, graduates of the University of Maryland School of Law. Summer research support from Dean Donald G. Gifford and is also deeply appreciated.

that in our "aging society" greater attention must be paid to older people with developmental disabilities, a group that has been exposed to many human rights violations in the past.

I. From Grotesque History to the Drive for Integration

The field of developmental disabilities has come a long way from the grotesque history of rejection and "untouchability" to the contemporary drive for integration and inclusion of persons with developmental disabilities in typical community settings. Along the way, Jeffersonian principles of human rights and human innovations were at times forgotten. On the walls of Jefferson's monument in Washington are etched these watchwords: "Laws and institutions must go hand-in-hand with the progress of the human mind as that becomes more developed, more enlightened, as new discoveries are made and new truths discovered, and manners and opinions change. With the change of circumstances, institutions must advance also to keep pace with the times" (Clinton, 1993).

Sadly, American institutions for the cognitively disabled failed to do that. Right up to the pre-World War II period, doctors and other leaders in the mental retardation field urged "total institutionalization." For example, a 1907 Wyoming statute expressed that very purpose, creating an institution Afor *all* feeble-minded and epileptic persons over the age of six.

Leaders in the profession fell into step and loudly supported this custodial approach. For instance, Dr. Martin W. Barr, M.D., an Easterner and president over 100 years ago of what was then known as the American Association for the Study of the Feeble Minded (now reincarnated as the American Association on Mental Retardation) called for the total institutionalization of all people with feeble minds.

In segregationist terms, Dr. Barr asserted a professional "consensus that abandons the hope long cherished of a return of the imbecile to the world." Instead, he urged legislators and colleagues to quarantine the people then labeled as "defectives" with these words:

> I think we need ... to convince the world that by permanent segregation only is the imbecile to be safeguarded from certain deterioration and society from degradation, contamination, and increase of a pernicious element....
>
> An ideal spot might be found — either on one of the newly acquired islands, the unoccupied lands of the Atlantic seaboard, or the far West which, under proper regulations, could be made a true haven of irresponsibility, and deriving its population as it would from the trained workers from the institutions throughout the country, might become in time almost, if not entirely, self-sustaining (quoted in Trent, 1994, pp. 142-143).

If Dr. Barr's dark vision had prevailed, western states and Puerto Rico would have become reservations for the "graduates" of the asylums for the feeble-minded. Besides a shutting away of all the "feeble-minded," the field at that time also called for involuntary sterilization of the "unfit." This policy of eugenics was endorsed in the infamous U.S. Supreme Court decision of *Buck v. Bell* (1927). In time, thirty states adopted involuntary sterilization laws and over 70,000 persons fell victim to those degrading operations. Even in Sweden, a country that has long prided itself on its humane approaches toward persons with disabilities, a 1997 study revealed that 62,000 Swedes were sterilized against their will — some because they had learning disabilities, some because they were not of Nordic stock. In one case, it was because a woman=s poor eyesight and inability to read the blackboard as a school child was mistaken for retardation. And this practice only stopped in 1974. Such human rights abuses were of global and historic proportions. For instance, Japanese authorities were responsible for the involuntary sterilization of more than 16,000 women in mental retardation institutions, with some of these operations occurring as recently as 1995. And on U.S. shores, a Cornell Medical School professor writing in the *American Journal of Psychiatry* in 1941, recommended that "hopelessly unfit children — nature's mistakes — should be killed, and the less unfit [sterilized]" so that "thereafter civilization will pass on and on in beauty." Was this medical educator unaware that Hitler had adopted a similar program in Nazi Germany in the late 1930s, leading to the slaughter of 300,000 Germans and Austrians dismissed as "unfit" and "useless eaters"? Or as Jay Katz, Professor of Law, Medicine and Psychiatry at Yale University put it, Athe Nazis began by killing their own 'defectives' and then went on to killing Jews and Gypsies, whom they also considered biologically "defective" (Katz, 1997, p. 5).

II. Human Rights, Ethical Foundations and Practical Actions

Out of such horrors, the world community resolved to recommit itself to human rights and ethical action. In the United States the founders had declared that certain rights are inalienable: that by right of birth, all persons are created equal and entitled to life, liberty and the pursuit of happiness. While this Declaration of Independence became one of the world's most influential statements of human rights and ethical principles, it brought little immediate relief to people of markedly substandard intelligence. Despite the early existence of these principles, persons with disabilities were not only overlooked for two centuries, but through acts and omissions they also suffered segregationist measures and other badges of inferiority. In the contemporary struggle to realize human rights for persons with disabilities, the advocate requires Job's patience and the faith to recall Isaiah's biblical question: "Lord, how long?" (Isaiah, 6:11).

RIGHTS IN ACTION

Putting ethics and human rights into action demands long-term commitments. The motivation to intervene to halt long-term suffering and deprivation can come from the attorney-client relationship or the ethical maxim "treat thy neighbor as thy self." Four cases handled by the University of Maryland's Clinical Law Office and the differences they made in the lives of four older clients illustrate this point. The first client, Charles Turner,* was institutionalized for 58 years at Maryland's Rosewood Center until his death at the age of 79. Charles labored for decades, six days a week, morning until night, without any pay. Clinic students and their supervisor discovered him during a class field trip. Eventually, the clinic won Charles a modest pension for his labors so that he could know that his life's labor had not been worthless — so that he could enjoy a few pursuits of happiness such as a vacation, gifts for his girlfriend, and a suit to wear when he received an award for his self-advocacy.

This labor practice — known as institutional peonage, or as involuntary servitude outside of institutions — was not unique to Charles. In 1988, the U.S. Supreme Court considered the case of two men in their sixties with IQs of 67 and 60 who lived in squalid conditions and in poor health on a dairy farm. There they received no pay and were isolated from the rest of the world. The farmer threatened these two men with reinstitutionalization if they did not do what he commanded. The Court deemed this practice a type of physical or legal coercion sufficient to warrant a criminal conviction against the farmer for the offense of holding the men in involuntary servitude (*U.S. v. Kozminski*, 1988).

The second client, Agatha, was also institutionalized for over 50 years, first in Rosewood, then in a bleak inner-city nursing home. When discovered she was in custodial nursing care, even though in relatively good health for a woman in her 70s. The cruel irony was that she had landed at the nursing home 20 years earlier as a result of efforts to reduce overcrowding at Rosewood. The nursing home, however, was even more restrictive for Agatha than the institution. She was rarely allowed to go outdoors. As her student-attorney, who was and is the State's Superintendent of Police, would remark, our worst criminals are not treated that badly.

A third client, Jane, stopped walking because she was deposited in a wheelchair for years at the same nursing home. She stopped walking because no one let her walk and her muscles atrophied. When she was released to a good community-based program, she like Agatha flourished, walked, worked happily in sheltered employment, and smiled again.

Finally Peggy, also in her 50s, was committed as a teenager to a state mental hospital due to her epilepsy and her parents' inability to control her at home. She

---

* Charles Turner's story, with his permission, was told during his lifetime. The other clients' names have been changed to protect their privacy.

was sexually and physically abused for years while in that institution where she did not fit and where her real disabilities went untreated. After two decades of her unlawful institutionalization, the Clinic won agreement from the state that Peggy would receive active habilitation and appropriate treatment in a group home and day program for individuals with developmental disabilities. Today, Peggy enjoys a full range of services and supports, will happily sell you her potholders at a quarter a piece and will tell you about the art therapy, the trips and other activities that give her — at long last — a life as close to normal as possible.

These examples underscore the importance of sustained individual legal representation because society can not afford to waste and abandon even a single life. While each of these individuals had major medical problems, their larger needs were for social and human contact and for being part of a community instead of being shunned.

IN SEARCH OF COMPASSIONATE HEROES

Part of the outpouring of grief for Princess Diana following her tragic death is that she visibly reached out to touch the untouchables of our time — AIDS sufferers, lepers, the homeless, the land-mine maimed. The public seized on her, in part due to great yearning for care and compassion in a world where our establishments are sometimes seen as cold and distant. In her brother's eulogy he called her a "standard bearer for the rights of the truly downtrodden." Shortly after, the world lost a full-time champion of its downtrodden, one who also identified with the "constituency of the rejected:" Mother Teresa, Nobel laureate and diminutive giant.

Mother Teresa served as a model for an ethic of human contact. Her life was a reminder that individuals can ignite a spark for lasting good. The saint in the slums of Calcutta was an example that the caregivers working in the trenches and on the frontiers, sometimes without a lot of sophisticated resources, can mean the world to those people whom they touch. As the <u>New York Times</u> stated (Editorial, 1997), she "found the energy and time to visit orphanages, hospices, and rehabilitation centers, invariably lifting the spirits of destitute children and patients." In austere quarters, she gave people a refuge from the streets and permitted them to die in dignity.

The intellectual disabilities field has known its own exemplars of moral courage and saintly persistence. Niels Bank-Mikkelsen pioneered the concept of normalization and implemented it as an official of Denmark. Burton Blatt in over 300 articles and other writings thundered against human abuse and worked to alter the status quo of dehumanizing institutions and excluding schools. And Gunnar Dybwad (1999) continues to deploy his formidable organizational and rhetorical talents to put ideals of human rights into actions of positive change.

III. The Parker Case and the First Step to Integration

The march to dignity and integration for people in mental retardation institutions began with an unheralded step on what was once the American frontier. The Wyoming case of *Heryford v. Parker* (1968) proved to be one of the country's first modern precedents on ensuring the rights of persons with mental retardation. Decided by the U.S. Court of Appeals for the 10th Circuit, this case revealed the rigidity and lack of due process experienced by the residents of the facility then-known as the Wyoming State Training School for the feeble-minded and epileptic, and by the residents of similar institutions throughout the country (Cohen, 1997). The case is about a lost childhood and how little we valued the lives and liberties of the children and adults relegated to such institutions.

THE RIGHT TO COUNSEL

At the tender age of six, Charles W. Parker was committed at a hearing with a prosecuting attorney, a certifying psychologist and his mother seeking his commitment, but no one to speak up for Charles and his liberty interests. At age 23, he was released to his parents' custody and two years later was returned to the facility *against the wishes of his parents*. The Court of Appeals held that under 14th Amendment Due Process young Parker should have been entitled to legal counsel at his initial judicial proceeding. In 1946 when he was committed at the age of six, he, of course, could not have made an explicit waiver of counsel. But even when Charles and his parents together sought his release at age 25, the institution's gates stayed stubbornly shut. But on June 14, 1968 the court found that he had been unlawfully committed because he had no lawyer to represent his interests. As a sign of the power of judicial process, he was discharged to his parents seven days later, as the institution's record notes, "in compliance with the court's order." The institution's records contain no further mention of Charles and thus he seems to have stayed clear of any re-commitments. Freed from institutionalization he returned home.

ETHICAL IMPLICATIONS

The *Parker* opinion is worth studying for its ethical lessons. The Court of Appeals for the Tenth Circuit looked at the realities of incarceration and not to the benevolent intentions of his keepers. The judges contrasted treatment ideals with the child's world reduced to a "building with whitewashed walls, regimented routine and institutional hours (p. 395)." As the court explained, analogizing commitment for mental retardation to commitment for juvenile delinquency: "Where ... the state undertakes to act in *parens patriae*, it has the inescapable duty to vouchsafe due process," assuring Athat a subject of an involuntary commitment proceeding is afforded the opportunity to the guiding hand of legal counsel at every step of the proceedings" (p. 396). Unfortunately this rule of law was and is often still ignored in practice.

In this case, the State feared that retroactive application of the rule Awould result in wholesale release of inmates in the Wyoming institutions and like institutions all over the country" (p. 396). But the court countered by stating that such a review was precisely the reason for applying the rule retroactively, concluding that the absence of safeguards can result in "indefinite and oblivious confinement and work shameful injustice" (p. 397). Unfortunately, the cases were slow to develop and the feared "wholesale release" took years to materialize. Thus the promise of *Parker* as an opening for deinstitutionalization was initially unfulfilled.

But if the institutional walls didn't come tumbling down right away, that day would come in various parts of the country, and for various other reasons. And in Wyoming the institution has shrunk as all hands have turned to correcting conditions that might work shameful injustice.

IV. Legal Cornerstones to the Disability Rights Movement

Five years after the *Parker* precedent, two federal class actions shook the disabilities field with path-breaking decisions that in effect announced that the civil rights movement had finally reached America's largest minority, people with mental and physical disabilities. Now that the 25th year anniversaries of *Wyatt* and *Mills* have passed, it is time to assess some of their larger impacts. In these two landmark cases, courts ruled that citizens with disabilities have constitutional rights to habilitation, education and humane care — rights that are present and enforceable guarantees. These judicial declarations were soon followed by legislative and regulatory codification. Even more importantly, the changes set in motion by legal victories helped to galvanize a broad disability rights movement. Yet despite these gains, one can still ask how long it will be until such rights are truly respected and internalized in standard professional practice.

The *Wyatt* Case and the Way to the Community

On March 12, 1971, a federal district court held that involuntarily committed mental patients had a constitutional right to treatment. Under this opinion, the patients at Bryce Hospital were found to be entitled "to receive such individual treatment as [would] give each of them a realistic opportunity to be cured or to improve his or her mental condition" (*Wyatt v. Stickney*, 1971). Within a year, Judge Frank M. Johnson, Jr. had extended this precedent to forge a constitutional right to habilitation for the residents of the Partlow State School and Hospital, Alabama's institution for persons with mental retardation.

On August 12, 1971, when the class action was enlarged to include these residents, Partlow contained 2,204 persons under conditions of bleakest despair and overcrowding. Ironically those conditions might have escaped remedy by the court had the lawyers for the parties not gone to inspect Partlow as a possible site to transfer patients with mental retardation from the two overcrowded state mental hospitals which were the initial targets of the *Wyatt* suit. The plaintiffs' lawyers were shocked by what they saw, and sought to persuade Judge Johnson that every resident was there involuntarily and each had "a constitutional right to receive such individual habilitation as will give each of them a realistic opportunity to lead a more useful and meaningful life and to return to society" (*Wyatt v. Stickney*, 1972, p. 390). This they ultimately accomplished.

George Dean and his co-counsel for the plaintiffs soon realized that they lacked the expertise — legal and professional — to identify fully the rights violated and the remedies to be sought. The case presented a unique set of challenges: (1) from a judicial perspective it was a case of first impression; (2) it raised a host of factual issues that had never been adjudicated; and (3) it called for the creation of professional standards that the field had yet to produce. To declare a constitutional right to treatment was one thing, but to define and implement a measurable and enforceable set of minimum standards of constitutionally adequate habilitation presented far more complex tasks. At an early stage of the litigation, public interest lawyers in Washington had read of the case in The New York Times and offered to assist. Dean readily accepted the aid of these lawyers, jointly representing the American Civil Liberties Union, the American Psychological Association, and the American Orthopsychiatric Association. The Justice Department also participated to represent the interests of the United States.

With the expansion of the class action to Partlow's residents, it was clear that mental retardation professionals and their association would be needed in the ranks of the *amici curiae* (friends of the court). The author (then with the National Legal Aid & Defender Association's National Law Office) and a colleague from the Center on Law & Social Policy were dispatched to inform the American Association on Mental Deficiency (AAMD) (since renamed the American Association on Mental Retardation) of the *Wyatt* case and to enlist their involvement as *an amicus curiae* in devising appropriate standards and presenting expert testimony. AAMD convened a meeting of its Legislative and Social Issues Committee to consider this request, and as good fortune had it, Gunnar Dybwad was one of its members. Dr. Elizabeth Boggs and the New York State Commissioner Frederick Grunberg — later a defendant in the Willowbrook case who would testify that "regression after institutionalization" was "caused to a large extent by the Willowbrook regime" (*New York State Association for Retarded Children v. Rockefeller*, 1973, Tr. 636). Among the half-dozen members attending, Professor Dybwad and Executive Director George Soliyanis immediately grasped the significance of the request, and were outspoken in support of the AAMD entering what for the Association was an entirely new form of activity. Dr. Boggs, as a past vice-chair of the Task Force on Law of the President's Panel on Mental Retardation, was also an influential voice in the AAMD committee's deliberation as the members were swayed by the advocacy of Dybwad and the invited lawyers. The die was cast and the organized mental retardation profession entered the judicial arena essentially on the side of the residents, and not of their defendant keepers.

AAMD thus joined with the other groups in filing motions to appear as litigating *amici curiae*. The court agreed to this unusual status, which enabled them not only to file legal briefs but also to have the powers of a party in taking part in factual discovery and presenting witnesses at trial. When the court rendered its decision in 1972, it would prominently express its appreciation for what it described as the "invaluable services" performed by the amici (p. 390).

These services and the alignment of the *amici curiae* with the institutional residents proved crucial. In developing the *Wyatt* mental retardation standards, the author and his colleagues consulted with the parties, reviewed the professional literature, and drafted the 49 standards that the court would ultimately adopt in its remedial decree as minimum constitutional standards of adequate habilitation. In an extended negotiation held in Atlanta, Georgia, between the parties and the *amici curiae*, 45 of those standards were stipulated to by all the participants in a memorandum of agreement. The remaining four standards were contested by the Alabama defendants and became a focus of a historic three-day trial before Judge Johnson. The trial also provided the court with the chance to hear from national experts who would validate the standards as a whole and suggest additional remedial approaches. Gunnar Dybwad, the lead witness in that proceeding, would become the only expert whose testimony would be quoted by the appeals court that upheld the *Wyatt* standards. His testimony was not only influential but prophetic. In precise detail, he laid out the destructive and debilitating consequences of custodial containment. He explained that many maladaptive behaviors were due to neglect and not to mental retardation *per se*. This deterioration, he maintained, was amply documented around the country: "that individuals who come to institutions and can walk will stop walking, who come to institutions and can talk will stop talking, who come to institutions and can feed themselves will stop feeding themselves. In other words, in many other ways, a steady process of deterioration" (Trial Record, p. 24). He foresaw a future in which alternatives in the community would replace such institutionalization. "In the long run, I see no need for Partlow," he testified, "but if Partlow will exist over the next years, it will be to take itself out of business" (*Wyatt v. Stickney*, 1972, Trial Record, p. 26). The author had asked him if Partlow was complying with the standards of habilitation proposed in this case. Professor Dybwad stated that it did not and that conditions bore no relationship to such standards, and then further replied:

The situation which exists and obviously has existed in Partlow for a long time is one of storage of persons. I am using that word because I would not use care, which involves — has a certain qualitative character, and I would not even use the word, 'custodial,' because custody, in my term, means safekeeping. And, as is visible to the visitor at the present time, employees at Partlow are not in a position to effect safekeeping, considering the number of people they have to take care of; so I would say it is a storage problem at the moment (p. 1313).

With this testimony anchoring its opinion, the Court of Appeals for the Fifth Circuit upheld the right to habilitation and the power of courts to set minimum standards for the residents of mental retardation facilities. So influential was the decision in *Wyatt v. Aderholt* (1974) that 348 other judicial opinions have cited that case. Furthermore, courts have referred to the *Wyatt* trial court's initial 1972 opinion on mental retardation standards more than 215 times.

In many of the leading subsequent judicial decisions, Dybwad appeared as a witness. In the Willowbrook case, a defense attorney attempted to undermine the force of his testimony on the numerous harms inflicted on its 5,343 residents by eliciting that his doctorate was in law rather than some more conventional field of expertise. It did not work, however, and the court went on to use a "protection from harm" rationale to order extensive relief. After almost two decades of litigation Willowbrook would become synonymous with institutional horrors and be closed. In *Halderman v. Pennhurst State School and Hospital* (1977), Dybwad's testimony was cited for the proposition that outdated approaches in the field had stressed protection and led to a self-fulfilling prophecy of stagnation in which individuals rarely exhibit growth. But once transferred from "depressing, restrictive" environments, as he proved, people with mental retardation were "able to accomplish a great deal" (p. 1311). The court relied on his assessment that based on his experience in visiting institutions in 49 states, Pennhurst was one of the worst institutions in the country (p. 1303). His key finding expressed the consensus that its residents belonged in the community rather than in an institutional environment that was not conducive to habilitation. Thus, the court concluded:

Many individuals now living at Pennhurst could be moved immediately into the community and would be able to cope with little or no supervision.... All the parties in this litigation are in agreement that given appropriate community facilities, all the residents at Pennhurst, even the most profoundly retarded with multiple handicaps, should be living in the community. (Dybwad, N.T. 7-68) (pp. 1311-1312).

Not every case resulted in a ringing declaration of human and legal rights. For example, in *Kentucky Association for Retarded Citizens v. Conn* (1980/1982/1983) [hereinafter *KARC*], the plaintiffs attempted unsuccessfully to block the opening of a new, but isolating institution called the "Outwood Facility." In this case, the core question was whether as a matter of federal and state statutory law the doctrine of the least restrictive alternative required all persons with mental retardation to live within a community setting. The plaintiffs argued that it did, relying on the theory of normalization as the "common thread" in the testimony of Dr. Dybwad and progressive administrators such as Linda Glenn. The Court of Appeals for the Sixth Circuit, however, disagreed, concluding that nondiscrimination law did not prohibit all institutionalization and that for some persons with severe or profound mental retardation, placement in a "new, more modern institutional facility" could constitute their least restrictive alternative without offending the law (p. 585). The case did, however have some positive results. In addition to improving levels of care, judicial declarations limited stays to 30 days for persons with milder or moderate mental retardation, affirmed their rights to least restrictive treatment and release from Outwood where the interdisciplinary team recommended a community facility, and upheld procedural safeguards for nonvoluntary committed residents (*KARC*, 1983).

In *Lelsz v. Kavanagh* (1987), Dybwad, identified by the court as the former president of the International League of Societies for Persons with Mental Handicap, served on the plaintiffs' team of experts that had greater success. Based on their testimony, Judge Barefoot Sanders found that the conditions at the Fort Worth State School violated the U.S. Constitution, other federal laws, and a prior settlement agreement in the case. With the defendants' acknowledgment that they ranked last among the states in financial commitments to citizens with mental retardation, and the experts pinpointing legal violations, Judge Sanders found the state in contempt of court for its failure to meet agreed upon standards. These standards included physical therapy, safe feeding, toilet training, behavior modification, individualized service planning, and numerous other requirements bearing on safety, freedom from abuse and neglect, freedom from undue restraint, and medical care. Because these standards were largely based on the U.S. Supreme Court's somewhat narrow view of protected liberty interests as articulated in *Youngberg v. Romeo* (1982), the *Lelsz* case focused on the institutional conditions rather than on integration. Yet even within these parameters, the decision was a reminder that when rights which "should be secured by the ethics and decency of civilized society" are trampled, the law has the means to give rights legal effect (p. 832).

Through the various twists and turns of the judicial process, *Wyatt* has remained a beacon over the years as well as an ongoing implementation matter. As the first institution-wide case, it led to a dramatic increase in suits either patterned after it or that staked out new territory. As a leading commentator noted, *Wyatt* had "massive influence" on state laws, state regulations, President Carter's Commission on Mental Health, and the burgeoning branches of litigation in both the mental retardation and mental health fields (Perlin, 1994, p.190). In Alabama itself, the case had achieved slow but steady results. Although conditions improved as staff and facilities were dramatically upgraded, the plaintiffs have continued to litigate this case to ensure implementation of the standards and to press for additional transfers to community settings. As the institutional census continues to drop, Dr. Dybwad's prediction that the business of Partlow will be to take itself out of business is gradually being realized. In the meantime, the parties have returned many times to the judicial forum to protect the rights of class members who still experience abuse, nontreatment and excessively restrictive confinement (Herr, 1999).

THE *MILLS* CASE AND OPENING SCHOOLHOUSE DOORS

Peter Mills and his class action case truly helped to revolutionize special education. Peter was twelve and living in an institution for neglected children when his complaint was filed. For almost a year, he had been without any education after his exclusion from the fourth grade for being "a behavior problem." To compound his woes, he had not received a full hearing, an adequate review of his status, or any offer to enroll in another public school or private school. Nor was he alone in being in an institution and on the educational sidelines. Two of the seven named plaintiffs in his suit were excluded from school while in extended stays in a public mental hospital; and other residents of Junior Village where Peter lived were also denied a publicly supported education. The institutions for the neglected were themselves neglecting their charge's educational needs.

Peter's suit pointed a powerful and novel spotlight on that constellations of injustice. *Mills v. Board of Education of the District of Columbia* (1972) was the first adjudicated class action on the procedural and substantive rights to special education. It was also the first to hold that *all* children with disabilities have the right to "a free and suitable publicly-supported education regardless of the degree of the child's mental, physical or emotional disability or impairment" (p. 878, in decree & 3). Moreover, it linked two problems that heretofore had been treated separately: (1) exclusion from school by reason of disability, and (2) exclusion, suspension, expulsion, postponement, interschool transfer, or any other denial of access to regular instruction on grounds of discipline. As discussed below, this linkage makes the *Mills* case especially relevant to contemporary debates in Congress, the disability field, and in the general media on when and how children with disabilities can be disciplined for breach of school rules.

In the early 1970s, before the filing of *Mills* and *Pennsylvania Association for Retarded Children v. Pennsylvania* (1972) [hereinafter *PARC*], its companion case, over one million children with disabilities were not in school because of the schools' inability to fund and create programs to manage their disabilities and meet their learning needs. The cases of *Mills* and *PARC* and their progeny forced schools to find those children. It then required school officials to give their families notice of their rights to a publicly supported education, expand the continuum of educational alternatives, hire additional teachers in both regular and special education settings to provide students with individualized instruction in the least restrictive individually appropriate environment, and add ancillary or related services to enable them to be transported to and supported in schools as effective learners. For the child with a disability, no longer would access to public schooling hinge on parental begging for services and the discretion of school officials.

The affidavits of experts like Gunnar Dybwad were of decisive importance in winning special education an entitlement. In the motion for summary judgment, the plaintiffs in *Mills* had to show that there was no genuine issue of material fact and that they were entitled to prevail as a matter of Constitutional and District of Columbia statutory law. The country's leading experts responded to the first part of this task. They made overwhelmingly clear to the defendants and to the court that exclusionary practices were widespread, that children could be educated no matter what their disability or combination of disabilities, and that the excuses for not doing so lacked factual and professional merit. Dr. Dybwad's affidavit perfectly fulfilled that aim, and concisely described the irreparable harms that school-excluded children faced. He began by noting that exclusion only accentuated any behavioral or emotional disturbances: "Whether they are aggressively acting out or passively withdrawing, these children need the protective stabilizing environment a well-planned suitable school program can provide" (para. 6). Children in institutions had even greater needs for "the guidance and stimulation of a full scale educational program" (para. 7). In perhaps his most eye-catching passage, he condemned the part-time education so common in that period in these terms. To provide children in institutions with "two hours of instruction per week can only be compared to giving a starving child two meals a week. Two meals a week do not make a diet and two hours of instruction per week do not make an educational program" (para. 8). Even more than typical children, the children of *Mills* required "the guiding hand of a skilled teacher" to recover from the lack or interruption of their schooling (para. 9). In referring to the research findings and the policy statement of the Council for Exceptional Children, Dr. Dybwad summarized the authoritative positions in favor of including children with disabilities in public schooling as follows:

> No child can be deemed ineducable, no matter how severe his physical, emotional, social or intellectual handicap. To the contrary, it has now been established that the handicapped child has greater and earlier need for structured education than other children. To deprive him of this education means to make him a less adequate person, functioning below his potential, with greater dependence on others, less able to handle the social and vocational demands one needs to fulfill to earn a living, less able to handle the human relationships which are the essential ingredients for community living. Thus the harm springing from a denial of education accrues to the community as much as to the child and his parents.

This position prevailed in the federal court and produced national consequences. Counsel for *Mills* was soon besieged with requests to replicate or otherwise help to achieve this judicial success in other states. Within three years, law suits had been filed in some three dozen states. In 1975 Congress passed the Education for All Handicapped Children Act (1975) to ensure equal educational opportunities and a minimum national standard for the nation's children with disabilities. As the Supreme Court would later observe in *Board of Education v. Rowley* (1982), the Act (Pub. L. 94-142) codified *Mills* and *PARC*, guaranteeing a meaningful education consisting of personalized instruction and related services for each child with a disability. With the provision of such services, integration took two giant steps ahead. First, it undermined one of the rationales for sending children off to institutions since now communities would be required to admit children with disabilities to their own schools. Second, as in *Mills* (p. 878 in decree & 1) it adopted the stance that any placement away from a regular public school class assignment had to be fully justified as satisfying the child's educational needs in the most individually appropriate, integrated way. A parent dissatisfied with the proposed placement was now empowered to challenge it through participation in the IEP process, negotiation with school officials, and the invoking of elaborate due process safeguards that could culminate in an administrative due process hearing and then an appeal to the court. Thus, questions of appropriate identification, evaluation, and placement have now moved from the realm of test cases to everyday advocacy practice.

The impact of *Mills* and the consent decree in *PARC* continue to resonate in federal statutory law, and the cases of children and youth handled at all levels. Under the Individuals with Disabilities Act (IDEA) a new generation of well-educated people with disabilities has thrived in schools and gone on to college in ever-increasing numbers. In the reauthorization of IDEA in 1997, advocates relied on *Mills, PARC* and the Congressional legislative history that sprang from those cases to fight back efforts to create exceptions to the all-inclusive mandate of IDEA and to preserve its central principle of no cessation of educational services. In testimony before the Senate, that argument was expressed by the *Mills* counsel:

> If we are to avoid generating new constitutional battles that parents of children with disabilities will have to shoulder, we must retain the settled legal principle and understanding among special educators that the words 'all children' in the title 'The Education of All Handicapped Children Act' promises that all must be provided individualized education (Herr, 1997, p. 90).

Those battles continue to be waged as influential members of Congress attempt, thus far unsuccessfully, to weaken the Act for children subject to disciplinary measures or young adults with disabilities who are in special education programs while incarcerated. In those future skirmishes, the legacy of *Mills* will surely be cited for retaining the bedrock principle that "all means all" since all children and youth with disabilities must be educated. Thus, the testimonies of Gunnar Dybwad and other pioneers are still relevant to the controversies of today and tomorrow.

V. Community Supports and the Spread of Disability Rights

One Wyoming case is a model for alternative dispute resolution and a sign of how far the disability rights consensus has spread. It was facilitated by turning to a valued mediator and helpful outsider, Professor Peter Blanck. But more importantly, the willingness of all parties to fix what needed to be fixed and to deal with each other as problem-solvers proved critical in the movement to community.

THE *WESTON* CASE AND ALTERNATIVE DISPUTE RESOLUTION

Cooperative state officials played an essential role in reaching and implementing the consent decree in *Weston v. Wyoming State Training School* (1994). Bob Clabby, who was faced with a court summons three weeks after his arrival, took over his new duties as the Superintendent of the Wyoming State Training School (WSTS) with a mandate for reform. He came to his new position with an understanding and agreement with the Governor to focus on those problems that needed to be fixed and to fix them. Clabby reported that he quickly decided to work with those involved in the suit as Ahuman beings" rather than to assume a defensive posture.

As previously noted, WSTS was established in 1907 and had been envisioned in Wyoming's state charter in 1890. Under current law, its purposes include the "training, care and custody" of people with mental retardation (Wyoming Statutes, 1997). In the 1970s, WSTS had a census of over 700. By the time the suit was filed in 1989 there were 395 persons on the rolls. By 1998 that number had dropped to 137.

The *Weston* class action suit defined class members as Aall individuals with mental retardation currently at the Wyoming State Training School or are currently or may in the future be at risk of placement at the Wyoming State Training School, including youths from birth to 21 years, adults and senior citizens" (*Weston v. WSTS*, 1994, p. 1). A consent decree, effective March 13, 1991, was negotiated by the parties and approved by the federal court. That decree required that WSTS numbers be reduced to no more than 161 by December 1994. To its credit, Wyoming exceeded that target early and became the first state in the Union to satisfy the terms of a consent decree within the initially specified time frame.

THE CLASS ACTION AND ONGOING DEINSTITUTIONALIZATION

With the impetus of the legal action, deinstitutionalization continues ahead. The state anticipates a continuing trend of five to ten persons per year transferred from

WSTS to community-based settings. As of 1998, there were only two persons under age 21 in residence and new admissions had virtually stopped. The population is an aging one. Approximately 60% of the current residents are age 40 or older, and 15% are over age 62. "Individualization" has been the watchword in this process. Supports and placements have been tailored to the Adistinct and unique characteristics and circumstances of each class member" (p. 5). In order to accomplish this transition from the institution to the community, Wyoming created a broad range of community facilities, programs and support services including opportunities for independent living, natural homes, adult companion programs, shared living arrangements, specialized living arrangements, and small group living settings.

Individualized program plans were developed with time frames specified for transition to the least restrictive living environment and day program for each individual. However, all parties agreed that no discharge would be made just to meet a placement timetable if appropriate community alternatives had not yet been developed.

In this process, Wyoming has become a model for the development of integrated services for citizens with disabilities. All parties recognized the importance of first using generic or existing systems to provide services for class members and only adding new services when existing providers could not deliver them in "a timely fashion" (*Weston*, p. 6); (Blanck, 1992, p. 268). According to local observers, the settlement agreement "simply did the job."

As in other states, Wyoming is faced with the perennial issues of expanding needs and limited funding. It made the political commitment, however, to put more money into community services. The result was an impressive growth of care and supports in community settings. Community placements increased from 1500 to nearly 3300 in a seven-year period. Administrators continued to shift funds from the institution to community services by having the "money follow the client" as persons were transferred to community settings. This is evidenced by a recent $4 million shift from the WSTS budget to community services.

A 1995 report showed that Wyoming moved from having a low state ranking in the bottom ten states to being in the top ten in terms of community-targeted expenditures. According to Braddock, Hemp, Parish, and Westrich (1995), Wyoming ranked seventh in the country in terms of community services' fiscal effort for persons with developmental disabilities and eighth in terms of the highest use of small residential settings (1-6 persons). The *Weston* class action suit was clearly a major factor in the extremely rapid growth of community services and placements in this state.

Additional good news from Wyoming comes in the form of a drop in safety-incident reports and complaints of abuse and neglect to minuscule levels. There is a waiting list, but it currently has only about 12 people, and good faith efforts continue to be taken to eliminate it.

Furthermore, community residential providers are now paying attention to issues of seniors with developmental disabilities. For example, ARK Regional Services of Laramie is giving seniors the options of working full-time or part-time as well as offering more recreational and social opportunities. In its senior program housed in "The Red House," consumers are free to quilt, bake cookies, visit the Senior Center, or just do what any other senior citizens do — as much or as little as they want to do. More and more it is being recognized that there are greater similarities than differences between typical elders and those with developmental disabilities. Older adults with developmental disabilities need access to generic elder services such as housing, in-house care and adaptive services, just as any elder person does. Nursing homes increasingly are seen as a last resort and not usually the most appropriate setting for someone with a developmental disability. According to the WSTS superintendent, both advocates and administrators share a common vision of walking down a Wyoming town street to see what life is like for persons with developmental disabilities. In this vision, one "wouldn't see anything because people with developmental disabilities are doing the same things as others."

The Wyoming deinstitutionalization experience has shown that once all parties and networks get beyond a competitive stance, they can work well together. The legal experience in this state has been practical and not doctrinaire; outcomes have focused on results, not paperwork and the system has displayed flexibility, not nitpicking. Most of all, it has shown that persons — even those institutionalized 30 years ago — can and do live safely and with dignity in the community.

LESSONS LEARNED FROM THESE ADVOCACY EXPERIENCES

The rights revolution has occurred on both individual and class representation levels. Advocates have had to recall the ethical importance of doing good for their clients one person at a time, one class at a time.

In responding to the advocates' demands and the clinicians' and self-advocates' rising expectations, the field has learned what works on an individual level. It has learned that the Charles Parkers could live in freedom. It has learned that the Charles Turners didn't have to wait for heaven to receive the reward and dignity of real pay for real work. So too, Agatha and Jane now live in comfortable homes anyone would be proud to call home. Peggy enjoys freedom from abuse and a full array of activities that keep her happy and productive. On a class level, Wyoming has used several of its assets to achieve not only compliance with a decree but results which go beyond it. For example, people are seen as individuals. In addition, Wyoming has a warmth and intimacy lacking in some other places. It is an atmosphere in which things can get done informally and quickly by just picking up a phone.

Wyoming achieved a blueprint for change in the Consent Decree and Order, described as "the foundation in transforming Wyoming's system of care and habilitation for people with mental retardation" (p. 2). The elements of that blueprint include: 1) a Quality Assurance Committee to monitor the service's quality and effectiveness, review public policy, make recommendations, and be a credible forum for resolving disputes; 2) an ombudsperson to focus on individual rights and services for those in the community, and to investigate abuse, neglect, or service issues; and 3) a case management system that promotes consumer choice and enables those choices to be "informed." The decree provides a legal commitment to building a system that "shall provide services and supports to class members of *all ages*" (p. 6) including a recognition that persons with developmental disabilities, like the rest of the world, have a right to retire. This right is given expression through an individualized program plan that must include a retirement plan that "shall be developed for class members 55 years of age and over" (p. 8).

Finally, the Wyoming process has deepened a sense of shared responsibility. As stated by the Wyoming State Department of Health's overview of the *Weston* agreement: *"All citizens of Wyoming share in the responsibility to help citizens who have developmental disability to realize their full dignity as human beings."* These are not just idle words in this state. For example, when a Wyoming resident was discovered recently to be in an abusive setting in a West Virginia "special" school, the Governor within 24 hours ordered his own plane to bring her home and out of harm=s way.

VI. New Challenges and Constant Vigilance

Despite dramatic gains in human and legal rights, there remains a need for constant vigilance. Around the United States, and certainly overseas, there are still places with life-threatening conditions in which persons with intellectual disabilities are allowed to live. It takes a long-term commitment from those with credibility to bring about necessary and lasting changes.

Aging persons with developmental disabilities often present challenges and vulnerabilities. Many still find themselves in strictly custodial settings with a lack of recreation and a low quality of life. With the demographic trends noted below and growing waiting lists, problems may get worse if action does not occur now. In addition, some states viewed the recent federal legislative change that eliminated the annual review requirement for nursing facilities as a "license to simply 'write off' older adults with intellectual disabilities and not provide oversight, appropriate services and programs" (Janicki, 1997, p. 2).

More people with developmental disabilities are approaching the life expectancies of their peers. In this aging society, the good news is that life expectancy in the U.S. is now 77.1 years. In the general population, historically there is a high rate of disability among those age 65 and over, with the disability rate of this age group roughly twice that of those of older working ages (45-64). Currently, 38% of men and 39% of women in our senior population has one or more disabilities (Kaye et al, 1996).

Nationally, human service systems in general will need an overhaul in order to more effectively meet seniors= needs. Under existing Medicare regulations, for instance, a patient does not have the option of choosing a private fee-for-service plan in order to obtain service from better-known doctors or from specialists. Yet advocates contend that "older Americans may have problems finding doctors who will treat them unless they supplement what Medicare pays" ("Bill offers new flexibility," 1997).

There are, however, some rays of hope in the "shake-up" created by managed care. As *The New York Times* recently reported, hospitals now compete for Medicaid patients and therefore clients with developmental disabilities on Medicaid may be now more attractive patients to some providers. "With the advent of managed care and lower fees for doctors and medical services, patients with private insurance are not as lucrative as they once were. This has pushed private hospitals and doctors to court the Medicaid patients they once shunned, mindful of the government dollars such patients bring with them" (Lewin, 1997).

Lack of focused attention in the states on aging and developmental disabilities also creates many questions about what happens to the elderly who also have these disabilities. Where do they live? Who treats them? Do they enjoy retirement programs? Is their right to life, liberty and the pursuit of happiness adequately protected?

For older as well as younger people with such disabilities, there is no reason for complacency. As Wyoming's UAP director wisely questioned: "Given that technology exists to support people in community settings, what is the rationale for keeping institutions open? What argument leads to the maintenance of institutional settings?" (Miller, 1997) The answer is probably intertwined in matters of ethics, money, and commitment to traditional ways of operating. Consider the examples of New Hampshire, Maine, New Mexico, Vermont and Rhode Island, which have completely replaced their institutions with community-based services. In short order, eight states will be institution-free. Norway, despite its dispersed population, has adopted a similar community-centered policy.

Despite Wyoming's progress, the state still faces dramatic financial disincentives for community placement, especially for the elderly. For example, the state wrote its application for federal Home and Community-Based Waiver funds for support for elderly persons with developmental disabilities at a maximum of $34,000 a year in nursing homes but at only $10,000 for in-home supports. In contrast, the non-elderly served under the waiver do not face an individual limit and the average adult plan costs $48,000.

VIII. Conclusion

As the rights revolution matures, it must find ways to ensure that aging people with mental retardation are included in communities. As the national Arc has noted, Ain too many communities, mental retardation support systems and generic aging services are not prepared to accommodate the needs of older adults with mental retardation. Supports for retirement, when desired, are not available, nor are community supports and services for people with mental retardation with other typical age-related conditions" (Arc, 1998).

In contrast to *Wyatt* and other heavily litigated cases, the *Weston* case shows that rights can be realized with problem-solving rather than through polarized and expensive conflict. The success of its alternate dispute resolution strategy to dedicate resources for remedies not rancorous litigation parallels the words of Charles Sumner, a Civil War-era statesman, who urged the redirection of communal resources:

> Give me the money that has been spent in war and I will clothe every man, woman and child in an attire of which kings and queens would be proud. I will build schoolhouses in every valley over the whole earth.

As this chapter also documents, direct citizen involvement is a critical ingredient to set things right. For those fortunate enough to live in Wyoming, the *Weston* agreement is a practical outlet for that involvement. Its insistence that a class member's rights "shall be cherished, valued, and protected and actively promoted" is at bottom an ethical one (p. 6).

For those who live elsewhere, progress also depends upon the power of courageous individuals to put ethical ideals and legal norms into action. Such individuals can alter the lives they touch. One recent federal law should encourage people to serve as volunteers. The Volunteer Protection Act of 1997 shields volunteers from liability lawsuits if they commit negligent acts or omissions while acting within the scope of their responsibility. Some individuals never waited for such legal protection before they acted. Thus, Gunnar Dybwad visited institutions in 49 states and scores of countries and helped some of their administrators to see their business as taking themselves out of that particular business. In the rights revolution, he models the role of tireless voice of conscience. David Mitchell is an unsung member of a soldier in the volunteer army for disability rights. By day the Superintendent of the Maryland State Police, he and other students at the University of Maryland School of Law rescued from neglecting institutions the people portrayed in the case studies in this chapter. "There's nothing worse then being nobody to nobody," Mitchell explained in trying to shed some light on the perspective of some of our most forgotten neighbors. To him, they were each somebodies. A number of Rosemary F. Dybwad Fellows have also spread the rights revolution by traveling to other countries to study exemplary laws or practices, an international direction that is also a hallmark of Gunnar's career.

Each of us too must become, in our own distinctive way, a standard bearer for the rights of the downtrodden. Each of us, in our humble and modest way, can bring dignity to the destitute, care and concern for our brothers and sisters who are elderly and disabled. Each of us can seek out our state's Charlies, Peggys, Agathas and Janes and give their last years the full measure of life, liberty and happiness that was so sadly lacking in their youth.

Toward that point of peace the rights revolution aims.

References

Arc (1998). Position statement on aging. Arlington, TX: author.

"Bill offers new flexibility in Medicare, but at a price," *New York Times*, August 5, 1997, at 1, 17.

Blanck, P. D. (1992). AOn Integrating Persons with Mental Retardation: "The ADA and ADR," 22 *New Mexico Law Review*, at 259.

Board of Education v. Rowley, 458 U.S. 176 (1982).

Braddock, D., Hemp, R., Parish, S. & Westrich, J. (1995). *The state of the states in developmental disabilities*. 5th Edition. Washington, DC: American Association on Mental Retardation.

Buck v. Bell, 274 U.S. 200 (1927).

Clinton, W.J. (1993). Remarks at a Ceremony Honoring the 250th Anniversary of the birth of Thomas Jefferson, April 13, 1993, in 29 *Weekly Compilation of Presidential Documents*, April 19, 1993, at 577 (quoting monument's inscription).

Cohen, F. (1976). "Advocacy," in M. Kindred, *The Mentally Retarded Citizens and the Law*, at 592, 600.

Dybwad, G. (1999). "Foreword," in S. Herr and G. Weber (eds.), *Aging, rights and quality of life: Prospects for older people with developmental disabilities*. Baltimore: Paul Brookes Publishers.

Editorial: "The Model of Mother Teresa," *New York Times*, September 7, 1997.

Education for All Handicapped Children Act of 1975 [renamed as Individuals with Disabilities Education Act], 20 U.S.C. " 1400 *et seq.*

Herr, S. (1999). Advocacy for the aging. In S. Herr and G. Weber (eds.), *Aging, rights and quality of life: Prospects for older people with developmental disabilities*. Baltimore: Paul Brookes Publishers.

Herr, S. (1997). Prepared statement of Stanley S. Herr. In *Reauthorization of the Individuals with Disabilities Education Act: Hearing before the Committee on Labor and Human Resources of Senate*, 105th Cong., 1st Sess. 90.

Herr, S. (1989). Happy birthday, dear "Godfather" Gunnar (remarks delivered on July 14, 1989 the occasion of Gunnar Dybwad's 80th birthday).

Heryford v. Parker, 396 F.2nd 393 (10th Cir. 1968).

Janicki, P. M. (1997). Report to the Board of the American Association on Mental Retardation, regarding Status of Alzheimer and Other Dementias Working Group Activities.

Katz, J. (1997). "Human Sacrifice and Human Experimentation: Reflections at Nuremberg," Yale Law School Occasional Papers, Second Series, Number 2, 1997, at 5.

Kaye, H.S., LaPlante, M.P., Carlson, D., and Wegner, B.L., (1996, Nov.) Trends in disability rates in the United States: 1970-1994. *Disability Statistics Abstract*, No. 17.

Kentucky Association for Retarded Citizens v. Conn, 718 F.2d 182 (6th Cir. 1983).

Kentucky Association for Retarded Citizens v. Conn, 510 F. Supp. 1233 (W.D. Ky 1980), aff'd 674 F.2d 582 (6th Cir. 1982).

Lelsz v. Kavanagh, 673 F. Supp. 828 (N.D. Tex. 1987).

Lewin, T. (1997, Sept. 3). "Hospitals serving the poor struggle to retain patients," *New York Times*, p. 1.

Miller, K.A. (1997). Personal communication.

Mills v. Board of Education of the District of Columbia, 348 F. Supp. 866 (D.D.C. 1972).

New York State Association for Retarded Children v. Rockefeller, 357 F. Supp. 752 (E.D. N.Y. 1973).

Pennsylvania Association for Retarded Children v. Pennsylvania, 343 F. Supp. 279 (E.D. Pa. 1972).

Perlin, M.L. (1994). *Law and mental disability*. Charlottesville, VA: Michie Company.

Townsend v. Clover Bottom Hospital and School, 560 S.W.2d 623 (Tenn. 1978).

Trent, Jr., W. (1994). *Inventing the Feeble Mind: A History of Mental Retardation in the United States.* Berkeley: University of California Press.

United States v. Kozminski, 487 U.S. 931, 953 (1988).

Volunteer Protection Act of 1997, Pub. L. 105-19, 42 U.S.C. " 14501 *et seq*.

Weston v. Wyoming State Training School, C.A. No. 90-0004 (D. Wy. Oct. 14, 1994).

Wyatt v. Aderholt, 503 F.2d 1305 (5th Cir. 1974).

Wyatt v. Stickney, 325 F. Supp. 781 (M.D. Ala. 1971).

Wyatt v. Stickney, 344 F. Supp. 387 (M.D. Ala. 1972).

Wyoming State Department of Health, (n.d.) *Overview to Weston Agreement*.

Wyoming Statutes Annotated ' 25-5-103.

Youngberg v. Romeo, 457 U.S. 307 (1982).

7

On the Closing of Mansfield Training School

Robert Perske
Darien, CT

Fifteen years ago, on December 6, 1978, a volunteer organization sued the State of Connecticut. In a class-action suit, known as <u>CARC versus Thorne</u>, the volunteers sued the state for the way it perceived and treated some persons with developmental disabilities.

The state saw some of these persons as burdens in their own neighborhoods.

The state saw them as needing programs the community could not provide.

The state sent them away to live at Mansfield Training School.

For most of those fifteen years, the Connecticut Association for Retarded Ciltizens — now known as The ARC of Connecticut — engaged itself in a battle that tested whether these citizens belonged in a segregated setting like Mansfield or in the community.

During that period, The ARC utilized the talents of its 21 local chapters with 3000 members. It used the volunteer services of seven state presidents (Luella Horan, Quincy Abbot, David Warde, Barry Bosworth, Mickey Herbst, Diane Aubin and myself). Two tenacious executive directors (Tom Nerney and Peg Dignoti) kept us together — always moving forward. We were represented by three of the most principled and committed lawyers I have ever met in my life (David Shaw, Frank Laski and Tom Gilhool). The lawsuit represented 14 named plaintiffs, 859 persons residing at Mansfield, 839 persons Mansfield sent to nursing homes, and numerous persons still at risk of being sent to the institution.

Today the battle ends. Mansfield Training School is closed.

Editor's Note: On April 24, 1993, the State of Connecticut locked the front door of this now-empty institution. It vowed to never force persons with developmental disabilities to live within its walls again. Before the closing, a ceremony was held on the front lawn with a wide range of citizens attending — including Governor Lowell Weicker, government officials as well as many former residents and workers. This presentation by Robert Perske, a former president of The ARC of Connecticut, was one of several made before the key was turned.)

Please forgive us for failing to feel sad or nostalgic when we think about this place. Instead, we remember the agony of the parents that The ARC represented. For them, Mansfield was the only alternative the State of Connecticut offered them. For them, it was Mansfield — take it or suffer alone.

We remember the Department of Mental Retardation's budget: Eighty percent went for operating institutions. Only 20 percent went for helping persons to live in their own communities.

We remember the photographs of Mansfield that were taken by the United States Department of Justice, showing:

- Persons with twisted legs and arms due to the lack of physical therapy.
- Others shackled to wooden chairs with leg, arm and waist restraints.
- Long lines of people sitting in day rooms.
- Persons staring endlessly into space, or slumped over in their chairs asleep.
- Others sleeping on the floor.

One photo showed 20 adults in diapers lying on one vinyl-covered mat. Another showed gang showers and rows of toilets with no partitions. Some of the toilets had no seats.

I will never forget one photo showing a little child sleeping under a stainless steel bathing slab — the same kind one usually finds in a funeral home.

We remember parents pitted against parents. Some went through hell before deciding to send their child to the institution. Others went through hell trying to keep their child out of Mansfield. They longed for community services and supports.

Then came the lawsuit.

We remember battles with the labor union. District 1199 of the New England Health Care Employees Union fought for their jobs. The plaintiffs, on the other hand, fought for The Constitutional Rights of the residents.

We remember battles between parents and their adult sons and daughters. Some parents wanted them to stay put — for life. But the sons and daughters wanted to move into the community.

We remember Judge F. Owen Egan's 116 page "Findings of Fact and Conclusions of Law" that was issued on April 9, 1984. He found that

- the institutional environment was destructive. (64).
- there were environments "devoid of potential for meaningful human activity" (65).
- physical restraints were used to control clients as a substitute for programs (68).
- many residents were denied their privacy and basic human dignity (73).
- residents were routinely restricted — even locked up (74)

- daily activities unfairly conformed with institutional routine (74).
- 22 Mansfield employees faced charges of abuse (76)

The judge's findings reflected the bleakness and the idleness of the place — as well as its terrible odors of urine and feces in many of the buildings.

On the other hand, it was the judge who brought the battling parties together. He allowed his court to be a learning place. He got the many parties talking to one another. Thanks to him, all parties (except for the union) came together and signed a consent decree.

Thanks to that consent decree, the tenacity of The ARC (led for most of those years by Peg Dignoti), and the Department of Mental Retardation (led by commissioners Brian Lensink and Toni Richardson), we see people with disabilities now living full lives in our own neighborhoods. We see them working. We see them shopping. We see them in restaurants. We see them volunteering for good causes. We see them paying taxes.

We even see those with multiple disabilities in regular classrooms with circles of so-called normal students as their friends. We see new technologies showing vividly that the true intelligence of some people far surpasses the labels and IQ numbers we laid on them according to the wisdom of an earlier age. We are aware of a powerful grassroots movement of persons with disabilities and so-called normals called The Inclusion Movement.

Most importantly we watch people who once lived in institutions now organizing as People First of Connecticut. When they lived in institutions we spoke for them. Now that these self-advocates live in the community, they insist on speaking for themselves. They are doing it with the governor, with legislators, at town council meetings and in their own neighborhoods.

All these breakthroughs show that the state has indeed changed its perceptions of persons with developmental disabilities. So Mansfield closes — but another remains open.

Southbury Training School is a segregated institution like Mansfield. There are 910 souls living there. Southbury has an operating budget of 65 million dollars — not counting capital improvements and property values.

Must we go through 15 more anguishing years? Or will our new perceptions move us to do things differently? Can the parties come together again? Can they study this situation and come up with a plan more quickly?

While working in Australia, I observed how the State of Victoria closed one of its institutions. The state sold the property and used the proceeds to pay for the housing and support in the community for all its residents for better than ten years. Could that work here? With our fresh perceptions and supports, surely we can do something better than we ever did before.

So, today, we say goodbye to Mansfield, and we hope the day will come soon when we say goodbye to Southbury as well.

SECTION III

International Issues

8

People with Mental Retardation and Europe 2000
Comparing Cultural Trends and Different Experiences

Ann-Margrethe Brandt
Norwegian State Council on Education, Oslo, Norway

THE NORWEGIAN REFORM FOR PERSONS WITH MENTAL RETARDATION: INTENTIONS, MEASURES, EXPERIENCES AND FUTURE CHALLENGES

A comprehensive reform has been going on in Norway since 1991 to improve the living conditions for persons with mental retardation. Before I present the reform, however, there are some facts about Norway you should know. Norway, is a small country with regard to population – only 4.2 million inhabitants, but when it comes to area it is a lot bigger: 323,878 square kilometers.

The Norwegian municipalities (local authorities) are quite different. Population varies under 300 to over 450,000, with an average population size of about 6,500 inhabitants. In many parts of the country, the population is very sparse. There are today a total of 440 local authorities in Norway, and 19 counties.

Norway has been a stable welfare state over a long period of time. The national economy is promising and the rate of unemployment is sinking, at the moment it is 4.6%. The rate rises to 6.9% if you count also those who have temporary work initiated by the government.

I will now try to outline the background and the intentions of the reform, the implementation measures, our experiences so far and finally the future challenges we face.

BACKGROUND

In Norway, as in most western countries, the care for persons with mental retardation has been dominate by institutional care. In Norway most institutions were established later than in other western countries. In 1950 less than 1,000 persons with mental retardation received residential care in institutions. By 1970 this number had increased to more than 8,500.

Because the building of institutions started so late in Norway, the governmental aim at that time – a full institutional care system – was never achieved. In the 1960s a rising criticism of institutions in general made it difficult for the government to continue with its plans, and normalization was introduced as a new concept.

The principle of normalization was first formulate in 1959 by NE Bank Mikkelsen of Denmark, later more closely defined by Swede Bengt Nirje in 1969.

The definition Bengt Nirje in the later years has come to use reads as follows:

The normalization principle means making available to all mentally retarded people patterns of life and conditions of everyday living which are the same or as close as possible to the circumstances and ways of life in society (Nirje 1982).

Thus normalization means supporting people in community settings providing an opportunity "to live like others amongst others". It aims at reducing stigma through nonstigmatizing service arrangements and to eliminate infantilization by serving persons with mental retardation in an age appropriate fashion. Other names have also been closely connected to the concept of normalization: W. Wolfensberger of the United States and K. Grunewalk of Sweden.

The Norwegian Association for Persons with Mental Handicaps was formally founded in 1967 after a couple of years with preparatory work. The organizations claimed civil rights for persons with mental retardation and services based on the normalization principle, and for the following twenty years this organization work actively to influence public opinion as well as political decisions.

REFORM DECISIONS

It gradually became recognized that an acceptable quality of living conditions and the rights of citizenship are difficult, if not impossible to ensure within a long-term institution. Commitment to the normalization principle as a guideline for services is first mentioned by the Norwegian government as early as in 1966. The further development of the ideas of normalization led to increasing criticism of the institution-based system. This new understanding also provide a framework for reconceptualizing the community-based system. These insights coupled with a number of institutional scandals led to a decision by the Norwegian government in 1987 to dismantle the institution-based system.

In 1988 a provisional law regarding closing down institutional care and agreements for private care under the so called "County Health Care for Mentally Retarded" was adopted by the Norwegian parliament. The objective of the law is:

a. To improve and normalize the living conditions for person with mental retardation.
b. To adjust the situation for person with mental retardation in such a way that they can live an independent life and participate in a meaningful and active fellowship with others.
c. To promote the closing down of institutional care and promote alternative services.

IMPLEMENTATION MEASURES 1991-1995

The Norwegian reform for person with mental retardation is a comprehensive reform with a five-year implementation period. Implement living and the closing down of institutions is an important first step in this reform. The residential institutions are closing down on a permanent basis. The reform applies to persons with mental retardation, whether they have been living in institutions or not.

The institutional care program, which operated under the county authorities, was terminated from January 1, 1991. From that time the responsibility for all persons with mental retardation was placed with the local authorities.

All local authorities in Norway had a long time to prepare for the reform from 1987 when the government decision was made, until 1991 when the reform was instituted. During this period information was a central issue, directed to different target groups: persons with mental retardation and their families staff both in the institutions and in the municipalities and last, but not least, the public.

The Ministry of Health and Social Affairs, in cooperation with other relevant ministries, has drawn up guidelines for planning the reform and for its practical implementation. Separate plans have been made for approximately 17,000 individuals. Five thousand living in institutions, 2,000 attending day services in institutions, and 10,000 living with their families in the municipalities, many of them without receiving necessary services. All local authorities also made separate plans. In the end all the plans are incorporated in the budgetary and action plans for the communities.

The Ministry has also drawn up a time frame for closing the institutional care. By the end of 1995 all the institutions shall be closed down.

Naturally a reform to improve living conditions costs money. The local authorities plan showed that there was a need for extra funding. Extra funding has been provided over a period of five years over the national budget to meet the extra costs.

IMPORTANT AREAS FOR EXPANSIONS

Historically, services for persons with mental retardation have been organized under the health sector, whereas today it is understood that other services and supports are more relevant and important for meeting the majority of peoples' needs.

Nursery Schools. Although these facilities are in general underdeveloped and unevenly dispersed, most children between the ages of 4-6 with a disability are offered a place in public nursery school. There are very few below the age of 4 years old who attend however. Support to families with you children with disabilities is an important commitment.

Primary and Secondary School. Most children with a disability receive education through the public education system, although the organization of this varies considerably. The Education law requires that each child be registered in the home school district. The earlier special schools are to a large extent turned into competence centers, and the intention is to provide pupils with education in their home neighborhoods and in regular schools, regardless of degree of complexity of disability. Primary schools have both professional and administrative challenges in complying with the reform's intentions in order that each child can receive an integrated education with whatever personalized assistance is required. Education laws have also established that secondary schooling and adult education must be modified to meet individual needs.

Housing. The reform has focused extensively on housing alternatives. This focus is primarily a reaction against the unacceptable standard of living conditions in the institutions. Norway has long had a standard for what constitutes acceptable housing for people in general, and these standards apply equally to people with disabilities. Most of these housing options are financed through the State Housing Finance Scheme, providing reasonable initial down payments and loan arrangements. Local housing associations have a key role in administration, planning and construction of new housing, and distribution according to need. Certain housing options require personalized adaptations.

There has been somewhat of a tendency to develop "group" homes, or situations where individuals have their own room, but share common living areas. Both the Ministry of Health and Social Affairs and the State Housing Finance Scheme warm against this, because individualized supports can too easily be organized as in an institutional setting. What constitutes a "home" is more than just having a house. The challenges for local services are to meet the special needs of individuals, without disrupting the ambiance and privacy or having one's own home.

Employment and Day Occupation. For adults, the activities and roles one has during the day are central to "normalization" of lifestyle.

Some individuals will be able to find paid employment in an ordinary workplace with minimal assistance. Many will need ongoing support in job finding, on-the-job training. perhaps ongoing individualized job modifications and supports. Responsibility for day occupation rests with the local community, segregated 'workshops" previously organized under the county. are now transferred to the local level, and are being reorganized. The State Employment agency will continue to have a role, as it does with other unemployed citizens. Very few individuals with mental retardation have full-time paid employment in integrated work environments. Supports for employment in integrated work settings are few, and are poorly defined, in terms of purpose. method, and responsibility.

Culture and Leisure. Having cultural and recreational interests and opportunities not only makes life more interesting, but is also a major way of coming in contact with other people who have similar interests and thus represent a possibility to make new acquaintance and maybe establish new friendships. Local communities have the responsibility to make accessible to everyone a range of cultural and leisure activities. This responsibility includes not only activities organized within the public sectors, but also includes assisting voluntary organizations and informal groups to include people with disabilities.

Practical assistance by paid helpers, or new transportation options may be needed. A conscious commitment to integrated activities is important, in terms of settings, activities and groupings.

Health and Social Services. Although responsibility f6r local health and social service provision has been established at the local level since 1984, the integration of persons with mental retardation will require a broadened capacity. Many new staff will be added to the existing service system, as well as some service workers who are being transferred from the institutional system.

Some persons with mental retardation also have impairments, such as sensory difficulties, and may need specialist attention. Many have health needs that have gone unmet for many years, both inside and outside of the institutions. Some also have additional problems directly caused by many years of institutional life. Specialist services will continue to exist as needed at the region/county level. Especially the smaller local authorities may have need for specialist expertise for individuals and situations that are particularly challenging.

Local communities are trying many new ways to organize services, in order to avoid building up a parallel and segregated sub-system. Most important will be finding new Wars of defining service content, methods, roles, and needed competencies for staff, in accordance with the intentions of the reform.

EXPERIENCE BASED ON RESEARCH FINDINGS

The work with the implementation of the reform has been evaluated continuously. We have already had a considerable amount of research presented, and some of it has been used actively in the current implementation process. Soon the Norwegian Research Council will have a conference presenting new reports and also a book of articles that will be published shortly.

Some reports of researchers have shown that the reform has been successful. Persons who have moved from institutions have achieved improved conditions of living and now have conditions that closely resemble those of the population in general. Some live in ordinary accommodations while others live in small housing units that are linked to each other. Research findings show that self esteem and self-confidence has grown and many persons are more self-sufficient than they were earlier. We have also come to know that highly disabled persons who have moved from institutions have gained a better quality of life.

It is important to bear in mind that the use of resources has changed with the reform. Studies show that within institutional care, only 56 percent of funds were directly utilized for services for the user. Now 95 percent of resources are used for such services in today's open system of care.

Studies show that the municipalities have made good progress towards building up a comprehensive system of services, but they have not achieved satisfactory results when it comes to employment and spare time activities. Studies also show that municipalities tend to organize care services in ways that may lead to new segregated systems within the local community.

In its nature research is to be free and critical, and many of the researchers are not necessarily telling the government that all is well.

FUTURE CHALLENGES

The Norwegian reform has gained widespread public attention, both nationally and at local level. It has great significance, since it is one of the most comprehensive and legally established social reforms of our time.

We have not fulfilled the goal of the reform yet. We still have many challenges ahead of us, particularly in the field of creating adapted work environments and using supported employment models to a larger extent. We also know that we need to improve the cooperation between the different department and branches of the various services that have responsibility for person with mental retardation. One important area for cooperation of this kind is competence building. We need to integrate competence on how to organize and provide services with close cooperation between different professional groups into the training course of service personnel.

It is also crucial to us to avoid building up a new segregated systems at local level that may lead to settings reestablishing traits of the institution-based system.

THE ROLE OF USER ORGANIZATIONS IN SHAPING AND IMPLEMENTING GOVERNMENT POLICIES – AND FINAL REMARKS

The user organizations have gradually gained a strong position in Norwegian government's decision-making processes. The Norwegian government has recognized the right persons with disabilities have to be represented through their organizations at national, regional and local levels.

The organizations have an important role to play in the development of disability policies and should have an advisory role in all decision-making on disability matters. We have realized that through cooperation with user organizations, we have a better basis to make the right decisions. The rights of persons with disabilities to be represented in the government's decision-making processes should be fundamental in every democratic country.

A good example of this cooperation is the implementation of the reform for person with mental retardation. The main user organizations, the NFPU as mentioned earlier, was an important pressure group before the adoption of the reform. During the whole process of implementation there has, in spite of hard discussions on several issues, been a climate of dialogue and cooperation between the government and the organizations. This cooperation has been a necessary prerequisite for the implementation of the reform.

When the reform period ends, the full implementation will not be achieved within that time. A series of challenges will have to be met also in the years to come when persons with mental retardation in the population are no longer a special priority for the government. The organizations representing these persons express concern and prepare initiatives to continue the focus on persons with mental retardation in the Norwegian society.

MY PERSONAL EXPERIENCES SO FAR ALLOW ME TO BE HOPEFUL

We know that many already have obtained improved living conditions and a new and better every-day life. We have met difficulties; some of them we have managed to meet in a constructive way, some are unsolved at this stage. Many people – politicians, community planners, community service staff, teachers, neighbors and person with mental retardation themselves, to mention some – have learned a lot so far in the process. This knowledge will help us to cope better in the future. I believe we are on the right track.

9

Getting There
How Are We Doing Internationally?

Walter Eigner & Helmut Spudich
Lebenshilfe, Vienna, Austria

Over the last few years Inclusion International (as the International League of Societies for Persons with Mental Disabilities is now known) has been publishing a magazine on inclusion of children with special needs in regular schools, titled "Getting There." This seems to sum up elegantly the current state of affairs in our human rights efforts regarding persons with intellectual disabilities: There is no more question of *where* to go, as there was decades before, but there is "only" the question of *how and how fast*. We have gone through a century of struggle about this direction: From unbearable conditions (the huge and neglectful institutions that so characterized of many decades of keeping out of sight and mind those that we did not comprehend, much less accept); to unspeakable horror (writing and thinking about euthanasia in many countries, and finally, in Nazi Germany, carrying out the unthinkable deed); to the charity of kind souls; to the striving to improve "the handicapped condition" and medical and pedagogical attempts of healing, yet separating; finally to healing that lies simply in accepting and including people in our midst who for whatever whim of nature only seem to be different. Society has indeed come a long way from the beginning to the close of this century that overcame unimaginable human atrocities and suffering towards a global society that is based on the Declaration of Universal Human Rights.

It was the British woman Eglantyne Jobb, who founded Save the Children in the aftermath of World War I in 1919 and went on to draft the first Children's Charter in Geneva in 1923, who first made an explicit reference to the condition of children with "physical and mental handicap" or are "maladjusted." As Gunnar Dybwad, the lifelong advocate of persons with intellectual disabilities, has pointed out, with this charter the groundwork was laid for a clear mission towards the goal of inclusion. There followed, after World War II, the UN Declaration of Universal Human Rights (1948), the Declarations on the Rights of the Child (1959), on the Rights of Mentally Retarded Persons (1971) and of Handicapped Persons (1975), the Decade of Persons with Disabilities (1981-1990), the Convention on the Rights of the Child (1989), as well as many other declarations of intent and practice such as the UN Standard Rules on the Equalisation of Opportunities for Persons with Disabilities (1993) or the Salamanca Declaration of UNESCO on inclusive schools (1994).

While this may seem to some like wishful paperwork, or like the theory of some social utopia that is nice but of little relevance to the everyday lives of millions of people, it is indeed the result of concrete action, not mere words. Just as the words of the Children's Charter were written as a result of the hard, down-to-earth work of a woman who saw the needs of neglected children and acted upon them, so have more recent documents resulted straight from the dedicated, intense and lifelong experience of self-advocates and their families as well as advocates and professionals willing to listen to the people they work for. And at the same time, once in place, these documents have become the instruments of further change in many countries throughout the world. They have become the basis upon which to file suits in courts of law, the blueprints upon which to build and fight for social services, the moral principles with which to argue the case of persons with disabilities in the court of public opinions against uninformed or neglectful communities and governments or simply prejudiced neighborhoods. Indeed: Merely declaring principles is not enough — there is a much more difficult job, namely to relate these principles to reality.

In many ways what society has arrived at through this tedious struggle for inclusion and "full participation" (the theme of the UN Decade of Persons with Disabilities) is both a clear vision as well as a patchwork of reality. Take the example of self advocacy and People First: Back in 1978, for the first time a group of self advocates travelled from the United States to Vienna to participate in the ILSMH's world congress. Quite obvious parents, professionals and advocates were not yet fully prepared for this new, emerging voice of self-advocates. It took another world congress, in 1982 in Nairobi, Kenya, to really allow room in meetings, sessions and plenary presentations. This was the start of a continuous movement, which led to good examples and practice that inspired others around the world. It took 20 years and many heated arguments even among those of good will for the notion of self-advocates to be represented on all levels of the work of Inclusion International, where before we have spoken "for them" rather than with them. And yet, this development is far from being complete, from being there: it is still a process of getting there, internationally as well as nationally. But the process will continue, as self advocates have started their own organizations and their own conferences.

The same holds true for the strategic focus on the development towards inclusive schools. The world took little notice of that development when Italy back in the early '70s started to abandon special schools and institutions in favour of attention to special needs in the general framework of its school system. But because many countries had already set out on the path described by the visions of the declaration of rights of persons with intellectual disabilities, they eventually found themselves on the same road as Italy (and some other early adopters), slowly but continuously headed for inclusive schools. It is when this process picked up in speed that exchanges of experience took place, that information from what was happening in one town and one particular school surfaced some other place as a model of inspiration. Today, while we are still a long way from *being there*, we are nevertheless *getting there* inch by inch, with each new class that finds purpose in inclusion and building a small world in which disability of one kind or another no longer results in being handicapped or prevented altogether to live a normal life in the mainstream of society.

So we would call it a patchwork with a vision that describes how we are doing both nationally and internationally in our struggle for a decent way of life for individuals with intellectual disabilities. To be sure, for each example of excellence there are at least two examples of negligence to be found; for each person able to achieve a fulfilling lifestyle we will stumble onto others whose lives may be miserable to the point of unbearable. But here is where the clarity of vision plays a major role in our struggle: It is precisely because we know what can be done and must be done in good practice that we can strive to change, to advocate, to call upon individuals as well as those institutions who are responsible to change for the declared better which has been proven over and over that it is possible to achieve. Governments, service provides, neighbourhoods, employers and individuals can not hide anymore behind the cloud of "handicap," of blaming the person with a disability for their own fate.

The idea of competition, for a long time seemingly reserved for the economic world and in fact met with reservation from many active in the social field, is bearing fruit here: It is the competition of ideas and of concrete actions that today is bringing progress to our field. Where we know of better services, we can point them out and demand a choice from those responsible to provide these services. Competition is what finally forced schools to change – a system which has been notoriously run with little competition and similar to the fashion of state monopolies. But the small scale competition that was introduced by inclusive classrooms made people demand similar offerings in their home towns, and home schools has brought a long overdue change not just for individuals, but to the school system at large, and not just to children with special needs, but all children.

Here is where the need for networking and for bringing about systemic, not just individual, change and implementing the right policies towards *getting there* comes in as the central challenge we have to face today on an international level. Of course, progress will always come true because of dedicated individuals who will not cease in their efforts to improve another individual's lot. But those efforts will leave many burnt out unless they are accompanied by the change that takes place on the level of social institutions and the law. Affecting change at government level is not out of our hands. If people with intellectual impairment are to be included in the community, there is a critical need for more collaborative efforts between public and private organisations and with all levels of government. We can no longer do it alone. We must all work together. The habit of "exclusion" has many disguises, and we have to be careful watchdogs and determined change agents. Because if we do not act against abuse and discrimination, then we ourselves become part of the abuses and discriminations.

Through networking with others we can form powerful partnerships and coalitions. Our own networking must be inclusive if we are to achieve a useful information exchange and to build up our capacities. And we can share our triumphs and our heartaches. By sharing a common goal and by facing similar struggles we can each extend our energy, insight and enthusiasm to others, so that the reverberations are felt in homes, schools, work-places, communities and government offices.

It is in this context that inclusion becomes meaningful on yet another level: In forming cross-disabilites partnerships, as well as joining efforts with other groups and organisations dedicated to make the concept of human rights work. For too long, the parents' organisations especially on behalf of persons with intellectual disabilities, have been on their own with few ties to other organisations, like those of persons with (other) disabilities, or altogether different social issues, such as the advancement of women's rights or human rights in general. This is of particular importance to the countries in development. In most developing countries far more boys are being educated than girls. However, again and again studies have shown that the education of girls is one of the best investments available to developing countries. As they say in India, "if you educate a man you educate one person; if you educate a woman, you educate a whole family." Indeed, girls' education can help increase family incomes, it can help to free women from subjection and give them wider opportunities, it can lead to better child health care and fewer child and maternal deaths. It can result in better nutrition and lower birth rates. *And* it will certainly lead to better care for people with disabilities. We need to work together to make progress for women against the combination of cultural restrictions, gender-based violence, disabling and dangerous childbirth, and customs that deny women access to education.

Therefore, we need to form coalitions with non-governmental organisations that concern themselves with issues in the broader context of social justice and human rights. And, of course, we must also form partnerships with governmental organisations that traditionally have seen the growth of nations only in terms of the growth of the economic output of these nations. Some of these relations, especially with UNESCO, ILO, the UN Human Rights Commission, WHO and more recently the World Bank, have become vital aspects of the work of Inclusion International, to make the voice of persons with intellectual disabilities heard in places where traditionally little attention has been paid to their welfare.

Sustainable human development is growth with equity. If we want to serve people with intellectual disabilities well, we also have to commit ourselves to the broader goal of social justice. This will also help counter a development that is of concern to us: While much progress has been made, and maybe even more progress in the acceptance and full participation of persons with physical disabilities, those with intellectual disabilities sometimes tend to be overlooked. For instance, particularly in higher education the gap of understanding seems to be widening: Yes, it is "of course" possible to include "the handicapped," teachers and school policy makers will say — meaning those who are "intellectually" fit. In today's technology driven industrial world opportunities for those who cannot easily follow the speed of change and need more time are easily being pushed aside. And, of course, with a market place that leaves armies of people unemployed, the competition for any job is fierce. It is especially in this light that we have to improve our efforts to make sure that persons with intellectual disabilities are not overlooked and ignored.

Of greatest concern in this regard are the alarming developments made in the era of genetic research. Once more, in a subtler and more tempting way, perfect humans seem to be in the reach of science. "No more disabilities, no more illnesses." That is the promise and battle cry of genetic scientists and their financial supporters the world over. Once we discover the gene that is responsible for cancer, and the one for depressions, as well as the ones that make us heartsick and homosexual, there is no question that we will also find all the "horrible and misdirected" genes that bring about disabilities. But what's next? The lurking danger of geneticism is the fixed idea that human beings and society are all just the result of our "genetic baggage," and the promise is this: Get rid of unnecessary baggage and you will get rid of the unwanted aspects of the human condition. This simplistic thinking does great injustice to the greatest of all human accomplishments: To grow in the face of challenge and overcome the limits that we may have inherited. This is the real promise of the human condition, and it is one that millions of persons faced with disabilities have proven time and again, to the enrichment of all of us. To be sure, there are benefits to scientific progress and we all wish to see these beneficial developments that, among other things, have combated illnesses like polio and brought about many improvements in the quality of lives. But beware of the illusion of the perfect world, which can turn out to be a vision without mercy.

The fight for people with intellectual disabilities has been a social struggle against false assumptions about people with mental handicap, against resulting prejudices, against discriminatory attitudes and against systemic barriers. Therefore social policy making is an arena for everyone of us, not only for so-called experts. But we have to understand that the struggle for people with intellectual impairment is part of a broader social struggle.

As UNICEF states in its report "The Progress of Nations," the day will come when the progress of nations will be judged *not* by their economic or military strength, but by the social well-being of their peoples; by their levels of health, nutrition and education; by their respect for civil and political liberties; by the provision that is made for those who are vulnerable and disadvantaged; by the protection that is afforded to the growing bodies and minds of their children. We all have a stake in that struggle for social injustice and equality: *We must invest in each other's civil and human rights.*

10

Overcoming Challenges of Organizational Retardation

A Convoluted Approach to Addressing the Eye Care Needs of People with Mental Retardation in Israel

Richard E. Isralowitz, Ph.D.
Department of Social Work, Ben Gurion University of the Negev

Background

In 1992 and 1993, at the request of the Israel Ministry of Foreign Affairs with the backing of the United States Agency for International Development, visitations were made to the devastated region of East Africa, Ethiopia and Eritrea, to determine how Israel could help address somehow, based on its experience and knowledge, the overwhelming social and health needs there. By no means are statistics a substitute for first hand visual experience; nevertheless, the level of destitution that prevails there reveals that the region and its countries rank among the worse in the world in terms of under age five mortality; gross national product (GNP) per capita is about $110; the average life expectancy is 47 years; daily (per capita) calorie supply as a percentage of requirements is 73%; adult literacy rate tends to be about 24%; only 25% percentage of the population have access to safe drinking water; 46% of the population have access to health services which are extremely limited; only 19% of the population has access to adequate sanitation; and, more than 75% of the region's children do not reach the 5th grade level of education (UNICEF, 1995). From the perspective of eye care, the region has a blindness prevalence rate of 1.5% which is three times the World Health Organization criterion defining the condition as a significant public health problem (Budden, 1981); and, as much as 95% of the population over the age of 65 have been reported with cataract (Steinkuller, 1983).

Nothing was accomplished from the visits other than a few reports laying out innovative strategies for "quick impact program development."

Upon return to Israel however, specialists of the Department of Ophthalmology, Soroka Medical Center in Beer-Sheva (Israel), as well as social/community workers were queried about the nature and scope of eye disorders within the Ethiopian community in Israel. Particular attention focused on the elderly for whom eye sight loss can be a serious debilitating factor needed to facilitate the adjustment process to a living environment.

Without adequate Hebrew language skills to express their needs; a fear of venturing out of their apartments and immediate neighborhoods; a lack of knowledge regarding how to access public transportation and services; and, a fear of interacting with modern medicine and physicians harboring attitudes of prejudice toward Ethiopian people (see Isralowitz and Friedlander, 1999), it is understandable why many of the elderly would not seek out public services for their needs. This situation lead to the organization and development of a model program of eye care and community outreach to people in need through a mobile eye care unit organized by Negev Project Vision through the Department of Social Work, Ben Gurion University involving volunteer ophthalmologists and an optometrist.

Administrative personnel of the regional Kupat Holim Clalit offices (National Sick Fund) and the Department of Ophthalmology of Soroka Hospital were aware of the need for mobile outreach eye care services. Without 'marching orders' and resources from central Kupat Holim Clalit offices located in Tel Aviv, however, little, if any, initiative is taken at the regional and local level of health service provision. For anything to happen, leverage was needed on the Director of the Kupat Holim Clalit to endorse andsupport a cooperative working relationship with Negev Project Vision and Ben Gurion University. Such influence was found through Project Vision, Inc. based in Atlanta (United States) which assisted in setting up a mobile eye care unit in the northern part of Israel. Also, the ability to generate cooperation was greatly enhanced when a donation was given to the Department of Social Work, Ben Gurion University to provide eye care services to Ethiopian elderly. The prize of the donation, so to speak, was a new mobile eye unit and portable eye care screening equipment. With resources and influence, a 'carrot and stick' contractual relationship was forged between Negev Project Vision/Ben Gurion University and Kupat Holim Clalit/Department of Ophthalmology, Soroka Medical Center. The Negev Project Vision/Ben Gurion University mobile unit and equipment was leased to Kupat Holim Clalit/Department of Ophthalmology for its purposes in exchange for a few days of professional eye screening and medical follow-up services each month to special target populations (selected by the Negev Project Vision Director). With the permission of the donor, the target population was expanded from Ethiopian elderly to include Russian and Bedouin elderly persons as well as people with mental retardation.

Initially, the stigma associated with people with mental handicaps caused a degree of consternation on the part of the National Health Fund (Kupat Holim Clalit) and excuses such as "they are not our subscribers for service," "their needs are being addressed through other resources," etc. were used to find a way out of addressing the needs of this target group. Negev Project Vision (Ben Gurion University) clearly stated to Kupat Holim Clalit that under the existing terms of contract, it was the University's right to designate special populations for the two days per month of professional medical eye care screening service received in exchange for access to the mobile unit and equipment. If the University designated people with mental handicaps, then Kupat Holim was contractually obligated to provide services. In a rather heated discussion, the issue was brought to a head - Kupat Holim Clalit would provide eye care services to the mentally handicapped at the request of Negev Project Vision or it would no longer have the right to utilize the mobile eye unit and equipment for its subscribers of medical services. In the end, an agreement was reached and the screening of people with mental handicaps was so successful that Kupat Holim Clalit encouraged press coverage of the services provided at two residential facilities in the Beer Sheva area for its public relations purposes.

EYE CARE PROBLEMS OF PEOPLE WITH MENTAL HANDICAPS: A BRIEF REVIEW

A number of studies provide insight of the nature and extent of ocular disorders among mentally handicapped people. Among a sample of 260 children and adolescents with mental handicaps, it was found that there was an unusually high prevalence of severe visual impairment (25%), refractive errors (24%), squint (8%), and a number of organic ocular diseases (8%) (Kwok, et al, 1996). In a study of mentally handicapped patients, 59% were found to have one or more eye anomalies including strabismus, refractive errors and cataracts, corneal anomalies, nystagmus, retinopathy, glaucoma, and other eye pathologies (Aitchison, et al., 1990). In 1985-86, an ophthalmologist screened 221 patients, ranging in age from six to 81, at a mental retardation institution. Regardless of the etiology of the mental handicap or the patient's age, the screening showed a high level of eye disease in this group. Only 44 patients (20%) had completely normal eye status without errors of refraction; 40 (18%) patients had errors of refraction only and eight had presbyopia only. Patients with one or more eye anomalies or diseases constituted 58% (129) of examined population.. Cataract was found among 40% of those people with eye problems; 16% were found to have keratoconus; 46% were found with strabismus; and 13% were diagnosed with conjunctivitis or blepharitis (Prokesova, et al. 1990). Also, clinical examination of 298 adults revealed a higher frequency of ocular anomalies of all types than is typical of a group of non-retarded subjects of the same age. From this study it was also found that fewer mentally retarded had appropriate optometric care than the equivalent non-retarded group of subjects (Levy, 1984).

Methods

PROCEDURE

In 1998, Negev Project Vision staff contacted the directors of two residential facilities for the mentally retarded in the Beer Sheva area to determine whether mobile outreach ocular screening of the residents was needed. The response was positive and the cooperation provided in terms of preparing the residents for screening reflected a level of organization that exceeded that normally found among non-retarded populations receiving screening services. Clearly, the intervention was a service not normally available to the residents of the facilities. During 4 days of screening, 66 people with mental handicaps ranging in age from young adults in the early 20's to adults over the age of 60 were screened. Screening was conducted by the Project Negev Vision ophthalmologist and nurse. Staff of the residential facilities used a modified "quality of life" questionnaire to use with the medical examinations to learn more about those people who were screened.

RESULTS

A structured personal interview was conducted by staff of the residential facility and the mentally retarded clients to obtain information about quality of life. Based on a scaled response of 1 (poor) to 7 (excellent), the mentally retarded participants that were screened reported that their general health condition was quite good (M = 5.136; S.D = 1.276); and, their evaluation of life was very positive (M = 6.455; S.D. 1.628). Only 2 (3%) persons out of the 66 examined recalled having had an eye examination; yet, 16 (24%) reported that they had visual problems. In spite of the high probability of visual problems for this group, only 13% (8 out of 61) reported having glasses and 20% (12 out of 60) said they needed glasses. Other functional characteristics of those examined included: 51 (80%) said they could not walk in the streets by themselves even though the majority reported they had no visual problems; in terms of watching television, 92% reported this activity of which 22% stated that they were having visual problems; and, among the respondents (39), 62% (24) reported being able to cook for themselves; and 83% who do cook indicated they had no visual problems.

Examination of the subjects (66) found that: 21% (14) had no ocular problems; 41% (27) needed eye glasses; 12% (8) had a cataract problem requiring surgery; 21% (14) needed an additional examination at the outpatient clinic at the local hospital; and the remaining people could be treated on location without difficulty. The findings revealed that the number of retarded persons who had glasses or who reported needing glasses was very close to the number found in need through professional examination.

DISCUSSION

A visit to Ethiopia and Eritrea, as reported above, lead to an inquiry and response to the eye care needs of elderly Ethiopian immigrants. This action in turn lead to a response, albeit limited, to provide ocular screening and treatment of the mentally retarded in the Negev. In both situations, the responses of government and representatives of major non-government organizations toward addressing the needs of these people tended to be similar "if they were not accessing health services available at walk-in clinics then there was no need for outreach eye care;" and, "the Ethiopian elderly [and people with mental handicaps] are a lost group and attention must be given to priorities." Indeed, the two populations are different; yet, at least in some cases they are similar – especially in terms of ability to access needed human services and the fundamental attitudes and behavior of policy and program decision makers to make resources and services available. More to the point, a lack of language skills to express their needs; a fear of venturing out of their cloistered environments; a lack of knowledge regarding how to access public services; and, a fear of interacting in unfamiliar environments (Isralowitz et al.,1999), may be among the reasons why people such as black elderly immigrants and those with mental retardation (even with staff support) would not seek out professional services for their needs.

Ethiopian elderly and people with mental handicaps, are minority "out" groups in Israel. As such, the provision of special services, especially those that tend to be more than a simple basket of normal processes of intervention require the ability to influence decisions through tactics of leverage negotiation and bargaining. This tends to be especially the situation when human services provision reflects limited funding resources, staff burnout and turnover, and shifting political fortunes including the influence of orthodox religion on policy and program decision making. Does that mean services to "out" groups are not provided or there is a lack of concern among special interest groups and advocacy organizations? The answer is no; however, for a society that was built on collective interest of concern for the welfare and well-being of its people, there should be no misunderstanding, some people do not receive their fair share of the resources and that gap between those who tend to be more inclined to be the recipients of government largesse than those who are not seems to have widened over the past few years. In fact, many recent studies tend to show that various elements of society, from kibbutz residents (Isralowitz, R., 1998) to Bedouin-Arabs (Abu Saad, I. et.al, 1997), from immigrants to veteran native-born residents (Isralowitz, R. et.al.,1997) are pitted against each other in competition and conflict, prejudice and repression.

In the context of community and organization development, a number of issues seem particularly relevant to Negev Project Vision and its efforts. The first aspect is social support. Through the use of university social work students and community service personnel, relationships were developed with elderly and mentally retarded persons promoting their understanding of the importance of proper eye care including ophthalmology and optometry services provision that may improve their quality of life. Like other minority "out" groups, these people are relatively isolated from formal sources and channels of information, such as physicians and other professionals; therefore, they are more likely to be more influenced by informal networks of immediate care providers, friends and family as well as religious leaders.

Second, by creating a successful experience, in the form of eye examinations and the provision of eye glasses, a natural campaign for eye care was created through a network of people in support of the project goals. From previous research, it has been found that eye care services, particularly the provision of eye glasses, has a positive influence on the ability of elderly persons to function. For this reason, it is believed that there would be a similar outcome for people with mental handicaps, especially those in open residential facilities who have the opportunity to live and work in a rather normalized environment. Specifically, the services made available through individual and group processes of health and social work services show that persons with eye glasses feel better physically, are more able to address their personal needs, and are more inclined to interact socially with family and friends (Isralowitz, 1999).

A third aspect of the project, which is still being developed, involves the need for multiple tactics of community organization rather than a reliance on a single intervention. "Neighbor-to-neighbor, residential facility to residential facility appeals; publicity campaigns via print and other media [especially for the children of the elderly], brochures and posters, classes, and group programs need to be considered if successful intervention is to be achieved. Therefore, individuals who may be isolated from one channel of information, say low literacy, isolation or economic disadvantage, may be reached by another so that the aggregate effects of all may exceed by far the impacts of individual interventions" (Fisher, et al. 1992: 253).

Finally, it appears that much has been achieved by Israel in terms of facilitating the absorption of immigrants, including those from Ethiopia as well as improving the quality of life and care for people with mental handicaps in a relatively short period of time. Nevertheless, the purpose of service provision is to be responsive to the needs of people regardless of age, functional ability or other distinguishing characteristics.

Clearly, deficits in basic care such as services to Ethiopian elderly and people with mental handicaps exist but these populations are not alone in terms of needing models of community organization and advocacy that address unmet needs, such as eye care, through public health and social work services.

References

Abu Saad, I. and Isralowitz, R. (1997). Social Cohesion and Intergroup Conflict in the Negev: Jewish and Arab Attitudes Toward the Absorption of Russian Immigrants. In I. Light and R. Isralowitz (eds.) *Immigration and Immigrant Absorption in the United States and Israel.*, Research in Ethnic Relations Series, Ashgate Publishing Ltd., 95-116

Aitchison, C., Easty, D., and Jancar, J. (1990) Eye abnormalities in the mentally handicapped, *Journal of Mental Deficiency Research*, 34, 41-8.

Budden, F.(1981). Blindness in Ethiopia Report. Geneva, Switzerland: World Health Organization.

Fisher, E., Auslander, W., Sussman, L., Owens, N. and Jackson-Thompson, J. (1992). Community organization and health promotion in minority neighborhoods, *Ethnicity & Disease*, 2, Summer, 252-272.

Isralowitz, R. and Abu Saad, I. (1992). Soviet Immigration: Ethnic Conflicts and Social Cohesion in Israel, *International Journal of Group Tensions*, 22(1), 126-134.

Isralowitz, R. and Abu Saad, I. (1997). Ethnic Conflict and Social Cohesion among Israeli Adolescents Toward Russian Immigrants. In I. Light and R. Isralowitz (eds.). *Immigration and Immigrant Absorption in the United States and Israel.* Research in Ethnic Relations Series, Ashgate Publishing Ltd., 82-94.

Isralowitz, R., Rosenthal, G., Lifshitz, T., Madar, M. and Shabtay, M. (1997). Ethiopian Elderly Immigrants: A Community-Social Work and Medical Intervention to Address Eye Care Needs, *Journal of Gerontological Social Work*, Vol. 27(1/2), 167-177.

Isralowitz, R. (1998). The Israeli Kibbutz: Shifting Attitudes of Social Acceptance and Rejection Toward Immigration, *Journal of Social Psychology*, 138(2), 259-262.

Isralowitz, R. and Friedlander, J. (eds.) (1999). *Transition: Russians, Ethiopians and Bedouins of the Negev*, Research in Ethnic Relations Series, Aldershot: Avebury/Gower Publications Ltd., (forthcoming).

Isralowitz, R. and Abu Saad, I. (1999). Competition, Discrimination and Conflict: Perspectives on Russian Immigrants in the Negev. In R. Isralowitz and J. Friedlander (eds.), *Transition: Russians, Ethiopians and Bedouins of the Negev,* Research in Ethnic Relations Series, Ashgate Publishing Ltd., (forthcoming).

Isralowitz, R. (1999). Vision Change and Quality of Life in Ethiopian Elderly: Response to Eye Care and Social Work Intervention (article in preparation)

Jaffe, E. (1995). Ethnic and Minority Groups in Israel, *Journal of Sociology and Social Welfare,* 22(1), 149 - 171.

Kwok, S., Ho, P., Chan, A., Ghandi, S., et.al. (1996). Ocular defects in children and adolescents with severe mental deficiency. *Journal of Intellectual Disability Research*, 40, 330-335.

Levy, B. (1984). Incidence of oculo-visual anomalies in an adult population of mentally retarded persons. *American Journal of Optometry and Physiology*, 61, 324-6.

Light, I. & Isralowitz, R. (eds.)(1997) *Immigration and immigrant absorption in the United States and Israel*, Research in Ethnic Relations Series, Aldershot: Avebury/Gower Publications.

Prokesova, V., Kriz, S., Berg, L. and Halvorson, I. (1990). Ophthalmologic examination of the mentally retarded at a central institution, *Tidsskr-Nor-Laegeforen*, 110 (13), 1659-62.

Steinkuller, P. (1983). Cataract: The leading cause of blindness and vision loss in Africa, Social Science Medicine, 17 (22), 1693-1702.

UNICEF, (1995). The state of the world's children, New York: Oxford University Press.

Meeting the Challenge of Intellectual Disability
An International Perspective

Peter Mittler
Professor Emeritus, University of Manchester

Introduction: Some Global Trends

The field of intellectual disability has changed out of all recognition since the end of the second world war and will no doubt do so again in the next half century. Although the nature and pace of change vary across continents, countries and communities, no nation in the world can justifiably claim that the quality of life of people who have an intellectual disability is comparable to that of their fellow citizens. In general, people with intellectual disability, their families and the staff who work with them are a low priority, compared with other disability groups. Their needs tend to be overlooked and they are often the last to be considered.

Nevertheless, significant advances have been made throughout the world in recognising the needs and rights of people with an intellectual disability. This paper aims to highlight some of these changes and to identify challenges for the future.

Summarising world trends, a number of key issues and themes can be identified. Only some of these are discussed in this paper.

1 A human rights and values perspective, based on internationally agreed principles, reflected in a range of United Nations Declarations and Conventions, as well as UN programmes and initiatives.
2 A reconceptualisation and redefinition of intellectual disability in terms of the nature and intensity of the supports required to adapt to the environment.

3 A shift of emphasis from custodial and segregated services to supported living in the community, involving access to mainstream services such as education, health care, employment, housing, social welfare, leisure and recreation.
4 An increasingly powerful self advocacy movement working for choice, self determination and autonomy.
5 A concern for more effective partnership between professionals and parents.
6 Organisations of and for people with intellectual disability working alongside other non-governmental organisations at local, national and international levels (including United Nations agencies).

TERMINOLOGY

Throughout this paper, the term intellectual disability has been used in preference to other available terminology, since there is evidence that this is gradually becoming the preferred terminology for international dialogue (Mittler and Serpell 1985). It reflects solidarity with people with other disabilities, as well as with Disabled Peoples' International. In keeping with this trend, the International Association for the Scientific Study of Mental Deficiency recently changed its name to the International Association for the Scientific Study of Intellectual Disability; similarly, a number of scientific journals have also changed their names. However, the life history of any terminology is now well under five years before it becomes unacceptable either to professionals or to service users or both.

Particular exception is taken by people with intellectual disability themselves to the use of the adjective 'mental' because it causes or complicates the confusion which already exists between intellectual disability and mental illness (Cobb and Mittler 1989) and also because it is used as a term of abuse in popular speech.

The former International League of Societies for Persons with Mental Handicap, which initiated debate on this subject about 16 years ago, finally changed its name to Inclusion International in 1994. In the United States, the Association for Retarded Citizens has become The Arc — not as an abbreviation of the former Association of Retarded Citizens but as a noun. The Canadian Association for Mental Retardation became the Canadian Association for Community Living, largely as a result of pressure from its self advocates, while Australia has statewide voluntary organizations with names such as Challenge, Active and Endeavour. Fears that the public would not know the goals of these organizations because of their new generalized titles and that fund raising would suffer as a result have fortunately not been borne out.

Finally, the American Association on Mental Retardation Revised Classification (1992) has radically revised its classification system and moved away from a defect model towards one which emphasises interactions with the environment and the nature and intensity of the supports needed by an individual.

Key Issues for the Future

SELF-ADVOCACY

Self-advocacy is the resolute movement of people with intellectual disability speaking for themselves, demanding that they be heard, and insisting on their right to make decisions. Self advocacy is beginning to have a major impact on planners, legislators, professionals, parents and on society itself. It is a growing voice.

The growth of the self-advocacy movement is summarised by Dybwad in the following words:

> People with intellectual impairments have – *in my lifetime* – gone from 'feeble-minded patients' to empowered agents of social change. They work to make the world a better place not just for themselves but for the rest of the world (Dybwad, 1996, p. 16).

The spirit of this movement is captured in the words of Barb Goode, a Canadian self-advocate and an elected member of the executive council of Inclusion International. Speaking to the full General Assembly of the United Nations in the session commemorating the end of the Decade of Disabled Persons in 1992, Goode declared:

> I speak on behalf of persons with mental handicap. We are people first and only secondly do we have a mental handicap.
>
> We want to push our rights forward and we want to let other people know that we are here. We want to explain to our fellow human beings that we can live and work in our communities. We want to show that we have rights and responsibilities.
>
> Our voice may be a new one to many of you but you had better get used to hearing it. Many of us still have to learn how to speak up. Many of you still have to learn how to listen to understand us.
>
> We need people who have faith in us. You have to understand that we, like you, do not want to live in institutions. We want to live and work in our communities. We count on your support to people with mental handicap and their families. We count on your support to ILSMH and its member associations.
>
> Above all, we demand that you give us the right to make choices and decisions rewarding our own lives (quoted in Mittler 1996).

Inclusion International now sees itself as a human rights and advocacy organisation. It directly confronts governments whenever there is evidence of abuse of human rights of people with intellectual disability. It has protested to governments on conditions in residential institutions and on the compulsory sterilisation of intellectually disabled people and has also influenced the wording of UNESCO's statement on the ethical implications of the human genome project, genetic screening and selective abortion. Together with Rehabilitation International and other non-governmental organizations it lobbies the United Nations agencies to promote the rights and needs of people with intellectual disabilities and plays an active role in the monitoring of the Standard Rules on the Equalisation of Opportunities for Persons with Disabilities.

MOVING TOWARDS INCLUSION

The principle of inclusion follows naturally from self-advocacy and advocacy for human rights. People with intellectual disability are demanding the right and the necessary support to participate fully in society and its institutions in the fields of education, housing, employment, public transport, health and recreation and leisure. Moreover, they want to participate in these activities together with their fellow citizens rather than in or from segregated specialised environments.

Children with intellectual disability are increasingly placed directly into an ordinary class of a mainstream school but with the individually tailored support of a teacher or classroom assistant (eg UNESCO 1995, 1996; Jenkinson 1996). To make inclusion possible for children with intellectual disability, the curriculum of the ordinary school needs to be made more accessible and relevant for all children (see Sebba and Ainscow (1995) and Chaudhury, Menon-Sen and Zinkin (1995) for international examples of good inclusive practice).

For example, the Peoples Republic of China has recently launched a five year plan to bring more than 3 million disabled children into ordinary schools, most of whom will attend regular classes, with appropriate levels of support (Lewis et al, 1997). Over a million teachers are being trained for new responsibilities. Other countries in the Asian region who are moving in the same direction include Bangladesh, India, Laos, Thailand and Vietnam (Mitchell and Chen 1996). Hong Kong too has launched a small pilot study involving nine schools (Mittler 1998).

SUPPORTING FAMILIES

Although the family plays the most important part in the life of the person with an intellectual disability, professionals around the world do not have a good track record in working in partnership with families. A major task for the next century is for families and professionals to evolve new patterns of working together which are based on principles of equality and partnership and which, at the same time, involve the intellectually disabled individual in discussion and decision making at every turn.

Families around the world have long been dissatisfied with the quality of the support which they have received. They are not satisfied with the information made available to them, the attitudes of professionals and the labels which these professionals often attach to families, such as "over-protective" or "rejecting". Families complain about the absence of partnership and equality in decision making concerning their children and how these decisions affect the family as a whole (Mittler and Mittler 1994).

For the past 50 years, families with intellectually disabled members have organised themselves to provide support for one another, to lobby for services and, where these efforts have failed, to establish services themselves.

COMMUNITY BASED REHABILITATON

From a global perspective, the vast majority of people with intellectual disability are entirely unreached by services of any kind, whether generic or specialised. Such services as exist are mostly in the larger cities and are commonly far too expensive even for those people who could access them.

The future for all countries but particularly for developing countries, therefore lies in community based rehabilitation (CBR). This approach trains and supports local teachers, health workers and others in the community to work together and in partnership with disabled people and their families. There is a long way to go before that goal is achieved in any country. But more countries are beginning to build links between CBR and education and there is encouraging evidence of positive results (O'Toole 1991; Helander 1993.

Conclusions

Looking to the future, we can discern a number of positive trends as well as threats. The growth of the self-advocacy movement represents a new consumerism which demands to be heard but it is a movement which is in tune with the parallel human rights perspective shared by many parents, professionals, and to some extent, by legislators and the general public.

The movement towards inclusion has been strong for some time but it is now clear that much more thought will need to be given to the development of a wider and richer range of informal as well as formal support systems. New thinking is needed on the nature of support for families and how to balance this support with encouragement of self-advocacy. Families need to feel empowered and supported in making real choices for their children while concurrently encouraging their children to become self-advocates and make their own decisions, even though their family may disagree with those decisions (Mittler 1996).

In the last analysis, all efforts to plan or provide better services and to meet the needs of individuals and of families depend on the support of the public and their representatives in decision making bodies at local, national and international levels. The education of the public begins with inclusive education which provides the next generation with the opportunity of learning and living alongside children who have a disability. But much also depends on the way in which intellectually disabled people are presented on the media and the way in which we use language to describe their needs (Shearer 1996). Family, social, cultural and attitudinal influences are critical in influencing the learning opportunities made available to people with intellectual disability.

Looking back over the past 50 years, much has been achieved through sustained and informed advocacy. But the goals for the next 50 years may be even harder to achieve in the face of continuing recession and budget crises and the lack of priority given to people with intellectual disability in many countries.

There is a clearer vision of the future we would like to see for children and for the families who will care for them for most of their lives. To turn that vision into reality we will need political will, reordered priorities and appropriate civil rights legislation that is implemented and monitored. In the last analysis, progress depends in large measure on empowered and committed families and above all on people with intellectual disability themselves being afforded equal opportunities to contribute to the communities in which they live.

References

American Association on Mental Retardation (1992) *Mental Retardation: Definition, Classification and Systems of Support* (9th revision). Washington: AAMR.

Chaudhury, G., Menon-Sen, K. and Zinkin, P. (1995) Disability Programmes in the Community. in Zinkin, P. and McConachie, H. (eds.) *Disabled Children in Developing Countries.* London: McKeith Press and Cambridge University Press.

Cobb, H. and Mittler, P. (1989) *Significant Differences between Mental Illness and Mental Retardation.* Brussels: International League of Societies for Persons with Mental Handicap (Inclusion International) (revised edn.)

Dybwad, G. (1996) Setting the Stage Historically. in Dybwad, G. and Bersani, H. (eds.) *New Voices: Self Advocacy by People with Disabilities.* Cambridge, Mass.: Brookline Books.

Helander, E. (1993) *Prejudice and Dignity: An Introduction to Community Based Rehabilitation.* Geneva: United Nations Development Fund.

Jenkinson, J. (1996) *Mainstreaming or Special? Educating Students with Disabilities in the Mainstream.* London: Routledge.

Lewis, J., Chong-Kau, S.J. and Lo, J.Y.C. (1997) 'Disability, curriculum and integration in China'. *European Journal of Special Needs Education,* 12, 2, 95-106.

Mitchell, D. and Chen, Y (1996) Special Education in East and South East Asia. in Brown, R.I., Baine, D. and Neufeldt, A.H. (eds.) *Beyond Basic Care: Special Education and Community Rehabilitation in Low Income Countries.* North York, Ont.: Captus Press.

Mittler, P. (1996) Preparing for Self Advocacy. in Carpenter, B., Ashdown, R. and Bovair, K. (eds.) *Enabling Access: Effective Teaching and Learning for Pupils with Learning Difficulties.* p.279-291. London: Fulton.

Mittler, P.A. (1998) 'Inclusive schools, effective schools'. *Hong Kong Special Education Forum,* 1, 2, 10-20.

Mittler, P. and Mittler, H. (1994) *Family and Disability.* International Year of the Family Occasional Paper No. 10. Vienna and New York: United Nations.

Mittler, P. and Serpell, R. (1985) Services: An International Perspective. in Clarke, A., Clarke, A.D.B. and Berg, J. (eds.) *Mental Deficiency: the changing outlook* (4th edn.). London: Methuen.

O'Toole. B. (1991) *Guide to Community Based Rehabilitation Services.* Paris: UNESCO.

Shearer, A. (1996) Think Positive! Advice on Presenting People with Mental Handicap. in Mittler,P. and Sinason, V. (eds.) *Changing Policy and Practice for People with Learning Disabilities.* London: Cassell.

Sebba, J. and Ainscow, M. (eds.) (1966) International Developments in Inclusive Education. *Cambridge Journal of Education, 26,* 1, 5-119 (special issue).

UNESCO (1995) *Review of the Present Situation in Special Needs Education.* Paris: UNESCO.

UNESCO (1996) *First Steps: Stories on Inclusion in Early Childhood Education.* Paris: UNESCO

12

Discussion on the Future Design of Residential Care for Persons with Mental Retardation in Japan

Akihiko Takahashi, M.D.
Toka Institute of Early Education, Tokyo, Japan

A worldwide trend to shift the basic principle for the care of people with handicaps from traditional institutional oriented programs to community centered philosophy was introduced to Japan in the early 1970s. For almost two decades, idealistic people in this field have been asserting that residential institutions for mentally retarded people should be demolished and be replaced by a community care program. Most people concerned agreed with this new idea in its theoretical principle. However, in a realistic point of view, parents' groups of people with mental retardation and direct care-workers in this field, and governmental officers are strongly insisting on the necessity of residential care for people with mental retardation. In addition, the real situation is that there are still more than 100,000 people with mental retardation who are "institutionalized" in about 1,700 facilities in Japan's 120,000,000 population. And the government is still planning to build new residential facilities for adult mentally retarded people in the future. This is a kind of big riddle in the welfare policy of present day Japan.

This dissociation of ideal and reality has resulted, and is still resulting, in long standing debates for decade on whether residential facilities are necessary for the care programs of people with mental retardation.

The "idealistic" group emphasizes the fundamental principle of the rights of persons with mental retardation to live within their own society and the right to choose where to live. They blame traditional residential facilities for its dehumanizing living situations and non-therapeutic conditions. Their thoughts goes to "community care programs" in which every problem should be adequately handled and solved by the network of social resources in the community. They often quote experiences in Scandinavian countries and blame the government for not following the Scandinavian policy.

Contrary, "conservative" group strongly emphasizes the reality that a) most residential facilities of Japan are small in scale (capacity of less than 60), compared with western traditional institutions and are keeping "home-like" atmospheres of living; b) most residents there cannot find the place to live outside the institution because their family, mostly parents, are already old and unable to look after them, and society does not provide the necessary resources to support them to live safely in the society. According to the "realistic" group, this lack of a support system in the community seems to be the greatest barrier to bringing people back to the society from the institutions.

This debate has been repeated almost fruitlessly, and parents' groups continue to ask the national as well as local governments to prepare more and more residential facilities for their retarded children. Their slogan is "Who shall take care of our children and where can they live after the death of their parents?"

There may be several reasons for such an endless argument. Among many, the ambiguous use of the term "institution" is one of the prominent reasons. Under the Welfare Law of Japan, the term "shisetsu" is used legally to mean residential facilities for mentally retarded people which is synonymous with the English version "institution". Half-way houses and group homes also are a kind of welfare provision for people with handicaps but are not called as "shisetsu" in the official terminology. However, unfortunately, the Japanese word "Shisetsu" in a general usage has a much broader sense and may denote public buildings such as a theater, station., bridge, and governmental office. "Shisetsu" means not only "institution" but other types of facilities such as a day-care center, workshop, group home, rehabilitation clinic, medical clinic, hospital and the like which can all provide services for persons with handicaps including mental retardation. Some people use the term "shisetsu" in the manner of a legal definition and insist upon absolute extinction of the traditional institution. Other oppose the use of the term "shisetsu" in the broader sense that includes different types of community resources, and contend that "shisetsu" should be maintained in the future, except for old-fashioned, dehumanizing institutions. In this sense, on-going discussions seem to fall into a rhetorical vicious circle.

In order to put an end to such endless talk, two study groups have started to plan the future picture of the system of care and treatment for people with developmental disabilities. One is a task force appointed by the Ministry of Health and Welfare which is to propose the future plan of total welfare policies for people with handicaps. The other is a research group, of which I was in charge, to figure out a program of care and treatment in both residential and day-care facilities for people with mental retardation.

The basic standpoint common to the two study groups isthat existing Japanese institutions have neither been the place of comfortable living for persons with mental retardation nor offered necessary therapeutic services for those with behavioral disorders. In other words, present Japanese institutions are not functioning effectively in order to assure the well being of persons with mental retardation. Those two groups independently have come to a very similar conclusion.

Their suggestion is to abandon traditional "shisetsu" in the limited sense, and remodel them into two types of facilities: dwellings for adult people with mental retardation and other developmental disabilities, and therapy oriented centers for person with challenging behavior.

"Shisetsu" as a Dwelling

This is the place for those who have difficulty in daily living because of maladaptive behavior or unfavorable conditions of the environment including interpersonal relations. The residence of this type is to provide the atmosphere of being respected and secured. There are no rigid time-tables for daily activities, training programs, or discipline to be forced to follow. This is just the place to live peacefully and safely for those who have not ever had a place of this kind even though living with their own family. It has been observed by many researchers and care takers that, under an unfavorable environment, people with mental retardation are inclined to show "maladaptive behaviors", especially when being kept in old fashioned institutions. Therefore, it can be said that some portion of behavior disorders could be the product of institutionalization.

The concept of the first type of residential facility is, at first, to eliminate pathogenic conditions in the environment which are responsible for maladaptive behavior of persons with mental retardation and secondly, to prepare living conditions to meet their needs and preferences. There are no special therapies or training programs, but living environments matched to individual needs and preferences which may have therapeutic effects on the residents. Residents may go out of facilities during the daytime to work or to have leisure activities. It is the way people dwell in their own home and go out to work or to enjoy entertainment out side of the home. The living facility is the place to guarantee "ordinary" lifestyle for persons with mental retardation. This can simply be called a "residential service". This type of residence may include a group home, care house, short-term residence, and an ordinary apartment house. There are no training staff, but it may need to be provided with supportive staff to manage daily living and care. When any kind of special support or treatment become necessary, professional support and help can be offered by agents or resources outside of the residence. Thus, facilities for work, leisure and intercourse with others as well as specialized treatment resources within the surrounding community of the residence should be indispensable to the first type of residential facility in the future.

"Shisetsu" as a Healing Center

As many researchers and clinicians pointed out, not all behavior disorders are the products of environmental inappropriateness. Recent studies showed that considerable portions of behavioral problems seen in mental retardation are either manifestations of dual diagnosis of mental illness and mental retardation or the result of psychosocial conflict. Those behavioral disorders cannot be cured by environmental remodeling and need specialized therapeutic intervention just as medical hospitals are for acute illness or emergency cases. Thus, these types of residential facilities for mental retardation shall be the places to give therapy for behavioral disorders. They should not keep "patients" longer than the necessary period of time for treatment, and should be provided in settings with outpatient sections as in medical hospitals. These have not been allowed by Japanese administrations.

Conclusion

Our conclusion is that we shall not go to the extreme of either demolishing all the kinds of residential facilities or preserving existing institutions in the future. Rather, we proposed two new types of facilities for mental retardation; the one as residential services to guarantee ordinary life within the network of surrounding resources of professional services in society. The other for therapy of behavioral disorders on both inpatient and outpatient services with provision for emergency cases.

This design may be common throughout Euro-American countries, but for Japan, it is the first time we have classified residential facilities into these two types in order to replace traditional residential care systems.

I close with a hope that our new concept of residential care systems can be the foundation for the future plan of care and support programs for persons with mental retardation.

13

The 'Lebenshilfe' in Germany

Tom Mutters

Foundation and Development

Not least among the factors which led to the foundation of the 'Lebenshilfe' in Germany – which has since become one of the largest and most influential associations for persons with a mental handicap in the world – were our contacts with Rosemary and Gunnar Dybwad in the 1950s. At that time Rosemary was in charge of international relations at the American parent's association, the National Association for Retarded Children (NARC), while Gunnar was its director.

During a meeting in May 1957 in the headquarters of the NARC in New York it rapidly became obvious that in Germany, as elsewhere, only the founding of an association like the NARC – i.e., a broadly based popular movement – would lead to a gradual improvement in the situation of persons with a mental handicap and of their relatives.

At that time the Dybwads already enjoyed international esteem in view of their work with mentally handicapped persons, a reputation which was to be greatly enhanced in the years that followed.

This is the reason why we should like to call to mind the beginnings of the Lebenshilfe in Germany – in order to honor Gunnar, an exceptional authority in international aid for the disabled, on the occasion of his 90th birthday.

The path upon which the Lebenshilfe set out in Germany at the end of the 1950s was rough and stony. We had to surmount many difficulties and with great perseverance. It was difficult and toilsome for us to have to set our sights on the next goal as soon as one had been achieved, but it was a challenge and we were encouraged by our successes. At one and the same time we had to overcome the devastating effects of a deeply inhumane political regime, relieve the plight of many thousands of handicapped persons, and free their parents from feelings of despair and resignation and from inactivity.

The beginnings of the Lebenshilfe really occurred six years before its actual foundation, in the state-run Philips Hospital in Goddelau near Darmstadt. Fifty-five mentally — and mostly multiply — handicapped children of refugees and displaced persons were living there as a result of a contract between the International Refugees' Organization of the United Nations and the Federal State of Hesse. They had been brought there from institutions all over Germany. Their parents had either survived the horror of the Nazi concentration camps or had been abducted from their home countries in central and eastern European countries as slave labor.

After their release they emigrated overseas, but had to leave their handicapped children in Germany, as at that time many countries forbade the immigration of handicapped persons. The United Nations High Commissioner for Refugees in Geneva had given me a limited mandate to look after the interests of those children — a task which was to give my own life's work an unexpected turn. The heartbreaking sight of those children, who spent their days dwindling and pining away in closely lined-up wooden cots, staring at the ceiling, some of them with their hands tied down, in a room stinking of urine and feces, starkly revealed the hopelessness of their situation.

Horrified at these conditions, I heard my companion (the deputy director of the hospital, a psychiatrist) say "You as a teacher are not going to turn any of these children into geniuses. Devote yourself to other things here, enjoy yourself while you are with us."

Nearly all of the children have died long since. But their suffering is inextricably bound up with the beginnings of the Lebenshilfe.

The moral of this episode in Goddelau and of what I saw there is the following:
Bureaucratic rigidity and arrogant and heartless attitudes and behavior towards weak and defenseless persons inevitably have a devastating effect on the quality of their lives.

If we know this we realize the real function of the Lebenshilfe, its most important socio-political duty, is to act as a watchdog.

Mental handicap, generally known in those days as feeblemindedness, was thought to be a medical but not an educational and social problem. So the feebleminded were frequently placed in institutions with the mentally ill, alcoholics and even with sexual perverts. As there was no medical cure, they were usually condemned to a life without any perspective, without any education or suitable means of occupation — almost to a state of vegetation.

Even doctors, to whom parents frequently turned for help and counsel in their distress, often recommended placing a child in a closed institution, reasoning that they would never do well anyway. A mother related in those days that her doctor had advised her to put the cradle with her newborn Mongoloid baby (nowadays we would speak of Down syndrome), on the balcony of her flat in winter, and that the problem would then take care of itself.

Attitudes like these, which were a protraction of the Nazi euthanasia ideology, were still present in the population, much more than is generally supposed. They were expressed with unbelievable and frightening candor in reactions to newspaper articles about the initial work and goals of the Lebenshilfe. Those letters starkly illustrated the situation of mentally handicapped persons and their parents in Germany after the Second World War.

At the celebrations for the first ten years of the Lebenshilfe, a quotation from Voltaire was placed at the head of a report on this foundation:

> A thing which is stronger than all the armies in the world is an idea whose time has come.

In view of the often indescribable plight of the children, and the despair and resignation of their parents, the time was quite silly more than ripe for the breakthrough of an idea for cooperative assistance. We knew from visits to and contacts with organizations in other countries, such as the USA, England and, above all, the Netherlands, that it was possible to channel such assistance. Pearl Buck, mother of a mentally handicapped daughter, (who later won the Nobel Prize) was an early member of the movement to found associations of the parents and friends of mentally handicapped persons, the NARC, in the USA.

Later, in her book *The Child Who Never Grew*, which was translated into German, she described impressively the experiences she had been through with her child before she was able to accept the fate dealt out to her.

On this subject she wrote:

> One must bear the suffering, one must know that suffering which one takes upon oneself contains its own gifts. Suffering has its own special alchemy. It can be transformed into wisdom, which brings not joy, but inner contentment.

In the early days of the Lebenshilfe, in particular, this book was close to parent's hearts. It helped many of them come to terms with their own experiences.

In articles in German newspapers and magazines, and in many press reports about the work at Goddelau, parents stepped into the limelight to ask for help for their children. One of these parents, mother of a boy with Down syndrome, tried in a newspaper advertisement to set up contacts with mothers in a similar situation. It was symptomatic that she received only one reply.

At that time the majority of mentally handicapped persons lived in the isolation of their own families without professional help, if they had not been placed in closed institutions. Many parents did not have the confidence to stand up for their handicapped child, they hid it from public view, let it go out in the fresh air only when it was dark and so on. They had often journeyed from one doctor to another, hoping against hope to find someone who could help. They clutched at every straw and put their faith in miracle drugs and therapies.

"Why me?" was the despairing question which they asked themselves repeatedly, without ever finding an answer which could help them lighten the load. At the end of a long and despairing search there was usually only the paralyzing realization that they were alone with their problems and that there would be no future for their child as for other children. In some, death wishes for their child arose as being the only solution. 'In this way I will spare him a life of suffering,' wrote a mother from Cologne. There were indeed cases in which parents, after years of unsuccessful searching for help, saw the killing of their own child as the only way out.

Prejudice, intolerance and overt rejection by an unknowing, uninformed society had at that time condemned the great majority of handicapped persons to a shadow existence on the fringes of society.

In an attempt to put an end to this situation, a group of parents and enlightened scientists met on November 23, 1958 in the Child Psychiatric Clinic in Marburg an der Lahn to found a German society of parents and friends of mentally handicapped persons. The invitation to this meeting contained, among other things, the program of the American parent's association NARC. It was decided that the Lebenshilfe should be an association of parents and professionals, and furthermore that both the day facilities mentioned in its program and its services (generally following Dutch patterns) should be owned and operated by the society as far as possible. For it was a bitter fact that neither the state, nor the established welfare organizations, were in a position to counteract the centuries old neglect of the interests of mentally handicapped persons and their parents effectively.

Factors which were characteristic of the Lebenshilfe were:

- Its structure was an association of parents and professionals running its own facilities;
- It had rapidly spread over the whole of the Federal Republic of Germany;
- The commitment of many of its parents and professionals, particularly teachers in special schools and doctors, but also persons from the fields of sociology and law;
- The acceptance it achieved, not only in political and administrative bodies, but also in the population as a whole;
- The gratifying interest taken by the media in the ever-increasing activities.

All this encouraged parents of mentally handicapped persons to publicize their problems, and also promoted the step-by-step implementation of initial programs.

A director was installed, at first in an honorary capacity, and from 1960, with the aid of the Ministry for the Family, with a salary. In the following years an increasing number of towns and districts founded their own local branches and eventually a head office was opened in each federal state of Germany.

The period of foundation was a particularly fascinating time, with a continuing series of successes. The Lebenshilfe was a close community of parents and friends of mentally handicapped persons.

A report from this era states: "the Lebenshilfe grew, it developed into a free independent nationwide society which awoke unexpected powers in the persons who became involved with it. 'We ran from pillar to post' is what it says in most of the reports from that time. 'We were always on the go, from office to office, from address to address, from family to family. Everything had to be done on the double, as it were, and the emerging self-confidence of the parents had an unprecedented impact on their surroundings."

The Lebenshilfe was weak financially, but strong on performance. At the beginning when there were no legal and financial means for the implementation of our program the tasks before us seemed insurmountable. However, we recommended that every local branch should start with playgroups in apartments or other rooms available and with a circle of volunteer helpers.

The fact that the Lebenshilfe was not contra but pro something brought it much goodwill from political parties and from the authorities. With their help, and the support of the media, but with special due to the elan of the founding generation at all levels, we had, after a decade of intensive build-up, achieved the proud figure of 350 local branches, 160 special nursery schools, 350 special schools for retarded children with practical abilities, more than 150 workshops for the handicapped, the first hostels, and about 50,000 members of whom about 50% were parents, and 50% were professionals and friends of mentally handicapped people.

Today the Lebenshilfe has about 550 local branches with head offices in each of the sixteen Federal States and with its headquarters in Marburg an der Lahn. It has 125,000 paid-up members. The legal and financial groundwork for what has been achieved has been done at the headquarters of the Lebenshilfe and by its councils and special committees.

The name of the Lebenshilfe (which means 'help for life' or 'help for living') is equally its program. It is a declaration of the inviolable right to life of mentally handicapped persons. Its goal is to give lifelong support, as stated in its program and this has not only been achieved to a large extent, but what is more, independently.

An important factor is that the costs for this support are, in principle, borne by public money (i.e. taxes) in compliance with legal statutes, but that the costs the branches have for running their own offices and other activities must be covered by their own funds (membership fees, contributions, etc.).

The Lebenshilfe cooperates with other NGOs, which have in some cases created systems of assistance. Its program, which is a guideline, but does not dictate daily practice, is the foundation for its cooperative activities. Aid for other countries, in as far as this is needed, is also contained in the statutes of the Lebenshilfe.

Over the years it has been able to exercise considerable influence on politics and on administrative authorities. It reacts to new developments in society and in knowledge concerning aid for handicapped persons, both national and international, with professional competence, while involving the handicapped and their parents.

The path it has set out on and its efforts to create a bright future for mentally handicapped persons and their relatives will not come to an end. The poet Friedrich Schiller described our work, in another context but very perspicuously in his poem 'The Ideals':

> This is the work, which is indeed slow, but which never destroys, which only shifts grain of sand to grain of sand to build eternity, but which strikes minutes, days and years off the great debt of time.

In the course of time we have been able to strike a piece off the debt of time owed to mentally handicapped persons and their families. But there is still much to be done and new challenges to be confronted, with the help of the handicapped persons themselves. It is becoming increasingly difficult to attract members of the younger generation to our work. But we should like to lay Seneca's words at their door:

Mihi crede, res severa est verum gaudium.
Believe me, a serious matter is a real joy.

14

The Situation of Mentally Handicapped Persons and Their Families in Eastern Europe

Tom Mutters

The decades of Communist dictatorship in the former Iron Curtain countries have had a devastating effect on their economic and social development, and thus on systems of aid for handicapped persons.

The rights of disabled persons, which were proclaimed by the United Nations in 1971 for persons with a mental handicap — and in 1976 for disabled persons generally — have been trodden underfoot in this part of Europe. It is true that before the political events of 1989 there were parents' associations in some central European countries, such as the Czech Republic, the Slovak Republic, Poland and Hungary, but they were in practice limited to organizing leisure time activities. As a result of the fact that these countries were only under Communist rule for a few decades and their cultural structure before that time was different from that in the Soviet Union, the circumstances of disabled persons there are more favorable than they are further east. The reorganization of the parents' organizations already in existence, multiple measures of aid from West European organizations, more effective processes of democratization and economic development, and, partly, support from other countries such as the USA and Germany, have contributed to the fact that the conditions for handicapped persons can be assessed more positively there than in the Soviet Union.

In other central European countries, however, such as Romania and Bulgaria, the situation can only be described as disastrous. A great amount of assistance has indeed been brought to these countries, but, generally, it has not been coordinated, and the majority of handicapped persons and their families still suffer from a situation which is unacceptable both from a humane and a social point of view.

The initiative taken by the Lebenshilfe in Germany, which was later financed in part by funds from the European Union for central and eastern Europe (such as PHARE, LIEN and TACIS) led to the founding of parents' associations in several eastern European countries.

Local projects in many places, supported by various Western organizations, aim to improve the situation. Trained-ships in Western facilities and seminars in the former Communist countries help to change and improve attitudes to mentally handicapped persons and to spread knowledge about means of helping them. Particular emphasis is given to the idea of helping parents to help themselves and to discussion about the public image of the person who has a mental handicap.

In discussion, parents, in particular, complain about the lack of interest the state shows in their children, especially outside the state system of institutions. Slowly some parents are coming to realize that they will have to take action themselves if the situation is to be changed and they are showing readiness to do so in localized projects. However, this is happening practically only in towns, and, there too, only in isolated cases.

So, despite the political upheavals in most of the east European countries, hundreds of thousands of handicapped persons are still vegetating, robbed of all human dignity, and under catastrophic conditions in closed institutions. Here mentally and physically handicapped children often lie naked, or clothed in rags, alone or with others, in old rusty beds on mattresses polluted with feces and urine, not infrequently tied down, and with shaven heads to prevent infestation with lice. There is practically no human contact. The few members of the staff are almost always persons with no training. There is no contact to parents.

Lack of nutrition, the often undefinable puree with which the children are fed, cold, and mental neglect lead in many cases to a premature death.

This kind of inhuman neglect can, with some justification, be called Communist euthanasia. More and more of the professional workers and the authorities in these countries see this aspect of the Communist past as being a disgrace to their country. However, they are completely without means to change the situation. Without trained personnel and immense material aid from the Western countries, thousands of handicapped children and adults will perish every year in eastern Europe as the consequence of privation and neglect of their fundamental physical and mental needs.

Western European governments, as well as the churches and organizations for disabled persons must not be allowed to register this gross disregard for the elementary human rights of hundreds of thousands of persons with handicapping conditions without taking action.

It is true that after the horror of the asylums became public, a large number of acts of assistance came in from all over the world, but, however much we acknowledge the magnitude of their selflessness, they are no more than the celebrated drop of water on a very hot stone. Even the program of assistance from the EU, like TACIS and PHARE, can only do little to make a real difference to the situation.

Under the system, the term 'valueless lives' was applied to mentally handicapped and mentally sick persons, a definition which was brutally implemented by mass euthanasia. But in Communist ideology, too, mentally handicapped people, being unproductive, were looked on as useless elements in the social system. They were excluded from society early on, while parents and professionals were forbidden to hold public discussions about their circumstances.

In professional circles in eastern Europe mental handicap was largely considered to be an insoluble medical problem. As a result, handicapped children were banished to mass asylums, often together with other undesirable and rejected children, without the necessary professional help. Even today it is not uncommon for the local authorities to try to prevent Western visitors and professionals from entering these sites of human misery. But what one is allowed to see is, compared with Western standards, bad enough.

It is true that in some towns in Russia there are homes which are relatively well equipped and in which the children are better cared for, but in most of these homes there are not enough trained personnel for individual work with the children.

We can assume that the better equipped institutions took in, either mainly or exclusively, the handicapped children of the party officials and of the priveledged bureacracy. Thus, as already mentioned, despite the principle of equality, some were more equal than others.

When they reach their eighteenth birthday the young people with handicaps have to leave the home in which they have experienced little advancement.

Only a small number succeed in finding a job on the general labor market. It is even more difficult to find a normal apartment for them. For this reason most of them end up in psychiatric hospitals or old people's homes, where as a result of the labor shortage, they are put to the care of bedridden patients or old people.

For the so-called children with 'mild retardation' children there were in the former Soviet Union, and still are, special schools, mostly boarding schools It is said that the children can be given better help in boarding schools and that this would avoid discrimination between children from the towns and from the country. In the boarding schools which were shown to foreign guests, the size of the classes was sixteen to twenty children. School hours were from nine till one. Social and physical training took place in the afternoons. A third of the children were girls. The children stayed at such schools until they were eighteen. The last two years were devoted to occupational training.

There were also so-called diagnosis classes for undefined cases. Here class size was eight to ten children. Their objective was to find out whether special treatment would allow the children to be reintegrated into the mainstream school system. However, as was reported, this hardly ever occurred.

The social insurance system in the former Soviet Union is today still characterized by a modest level of benefits, without a contribution from the insured, but also without the guarantee of a minimum income. The officially proclaimed principle of equality was never kept to in reality. For the nomenclature there was a complicated system of favors. Among those at a disadvantage in this system were handicapped persons and their families. However, so-called 'invalids,' and their families received a very modest pension, the size of which apparently differed in the individual towns and republics.

Only 'invalids' who are completely incapable of work and in need of care receive a small invalid pension. Everything else is left to the family. The miserable socioeconomic situation in Russia means that both men and women have to go out to work, the living conditions are extremely modest, (citizens of this country can generally lay claim to only 6 square meters living area per person), and the possession of a mentally handicapped child is looked on very negatively in the uninformed population. Consequently, children with mental and other severe handicaps are to be found at home almost only in the country, while in the towns many live in institutions.

After the political change in the former Communist bloc non-state organizations sprung up like mushrooms almost everywhere and the field of aid for the handicapped was no exception. However, most of them lack good financial footing and do little to attain their goals. Many of them do not have a uniform sense of purpose and all of them work independently of each other most of the time. Initially there were many such groups who blazed 'help for the disabled' across their banners, without even identifying the kind of handicap.

The catastrophic financial situation is another reason why there are no public funds for individual measures which are initiated. The small day centers which are started here and there by parent associations with aid from professionals are usually financed solely by their own funds and by donations. The commitment and the almost despairing courage with which these pioneers have, despite all hindrances, started to create a humane existence for their charges are highly admirable and deserve every kind of support from the more privileged part of our common European world.

"It is especially important," one of them, a lady doctor who has founded an association like the Lebenshilfe and a day center in Odessa, once said at a conference in Marburg, "to give parents the feeling that they are not left alone with their problems any longer, to boost their self-confidence, so that they can get up enough courage to step forward and say: 'That is my son, my daughter.'" Thanks to the activities of such parent's groups a slowly growing number of parents are beginning to produce this courage and to give up their lethargic attitude. However, the majority of them still assume a position of 'waiting and watching' because of the experiences they had in the former Communist system.

Recently, a father of a multiply handicapped child in St. Petersburg, the former Leningrad, where some years ago a slowly expanding parent's association was founded with Lebenshilfe help, said the following:

We were sometimes told things like this: "You can throw your child in the snow, it won't even catch cold. It will never be able to tell the difference between its mother and a nurse. I never asked you to give birth to a child of this sort."

The latter was the remark by a representative of an administrative authority to a poor mother, who asked for help for her child. No, our children are not loved in St. Petersburg, by the city which claims to be the leading spiritual and cultural center of our country.

In daylight a mother of 'such' a child will not dare to go out on the street; she only goes out after dark. She does that because she cannot bear to hear the remarks of the passersby. Many people think that the parents of such children are drunks or prostitutes.

We, however, the parents of mentally handicapped children, are extremely patient. We feel no hate towards these persons. Our feelings have very deep roots. Our former rulers tried long and systematically to annihilate our people spiritually. A slogan of the thirties was: "a healthy spirit can only exist in a healthy body."

This slogan meant that all those who were crippled in any way fell by the wayside, trampled on in the mud of heartlessness. Our ideologists tried to tell the world that our country was completely healthy. How much did the faces of our Mongoloid children contrast with this proud declaration! How much was this statement in contradiction to the healthy facade of a pure communism! Decades will pass before our country is reborn in mercifulness and kindness. At present our children are denied all human rights. Newborn babies have to live until their life's end as outcasts from society. The rights of mentally handicapped persons as proclaimed by the United Nations also apply in Russia. During the voting on this declaration in the General Assembly of the United Nations the former Soviet government abstained, as is well known. I should like to ask the present parliament to discuss this problem anew and to reach an appropriate decision.

The fate of our children is different from that of mentally handicapped children n the Western countries.

- *Our children are still called imbeciles.* Medical and educational commissions still only apply this negative terminology which does not indicate a child's potential. As a result the child is given a label: 'incapable of learning.' As soon as the child is included in the category of the mentally handicapped it receives an automatic entitlement to psycho-pharmacological drugs. It is almost impossible to protest against the judgment of such a commission but the label will accompany the child for the rest of its life.
- *Our children are considered to be of less value from birth onwards.* In all official documents they are defined as child invalids. 'Invalid' literally means 'of less value.' Do we need to comment on this?
- *Our children do not live they merely exist.* The powerful and the whole of society look on our children only as 'beings'. They have no right to dignity

and to a human kind of life. The state pays out millions of rubles for its members who are still in existence, but does not invest a penny for their rehabilitation.
- *The lives of our children are like a path into the void.* Along this path there are only two places of refuge for our children: the family, if their parents have not rejected them, or a state institution if they have one available.

  In the second case the way into the void is very clearly defined: from birth to four years of age it will be a baby house. Afterwards it will be a psychoneurological children's home, where they live until they are eighteen. The next step is a home of the same kind for adults, where our children are obliged to live until they die. In all these institutions, they can expect a certain amount of support, a primitive kind of work and complete isolation. It is like living on a desert island. In my speech I called these children 'our children'. This was no oversight. They really are our children, as only their parents love them. That is their social status in our society.

In the meantime, owing to the foundation of a parent's association with Western support, considerable progress has been made in St. Petersburg in the fields of counseling, pre-school aids, schooling and education and in initial work programs for a good number of children and youths.

Constant contact with the authorities and with the media, in this part of Russia has also played a role. In the former Communist system the intervention of radio and press was never taken into consideration, as it was alleged that the state always did 'everything that was necessary.' Now attempts are being made in several cities in eastern Europe to use the media to arouse more understanding in the population.

However these efforts often attract little attention. The difficult situation in which many people find themselves in these countries means that they have little time to worry about the troubles of others.

Emigrant families (families of German descent who have emigrated to Germany) who have a mentally handicapped child, and who mostly lived in village surroundings in the former Soviet Union, reported discrimination of their children by neighbors.

A mother who had given birth to a child with Down syndrome in hospital, received the advice from her doctor that she should leave the child there and she herself should, if possible, move to another town and forget it. Others report that information about the diagnosis was coupled with personal comments, such a "you have no doubt noticed yourself that you have given birth to a simpleton." There was no psychosocial support, say these families, and everyone was left to confront the situation as best he or she could.

A mother who now lives in Germany said: "In Russia our children were forgotten children, but here they are treated like human beings". In some families in

Russia handicapped children were, at most, tolerated. This meant that a wheelchair or therapeutic treatment were denied to the children even by their own families. This situation had particularly severe effects for more elderly handicapped persons, who are entirely reliant on the support of their families, as help is not given by any authority.

As mental handicap was considered to be a medical problem in eastern Europe, the results of medical examinations still form the basis for the classification of the children and their placement in institutions. Day centers for them are never a matter for consideration.

These days the diagnosis is generally given by a team of doctors and defectologists. The training the defectologists formerly received was basically medical. As a result the tests used in the process of diagnosis still usually involve an examination of the nervous system and observation of perceptivity. The tests are a completely insufficient basis for judgment, as they only give information about quantitative performance. Qualitative and emotional factors remain totally unaccounted for.

Parents were often told that their child would not be able to learn well or that it was feeble-minded and ineducable. In a period from 1990 to 1991 a team of experts from Poland made several visits to institutions for the mentally handicapped in St. Petersburg and discovered that children who had been diagnosed by their Russian colleagues as being mentally handicapped were, in fact, at the boundary to normal development. Some of the children examined were well aware of the disadvantage of their situation and had given a realistic assessment of their living conditions.

In the examination of young children the guideline was a special test for internal use, in which the developmental stages were defined for every week of life after birth. The requirements in these tests were so high that even normally developed children did not comply with them and were diagnosed as being retarded. According to the Polish teams, the assessment of older children was based only on conversations and a very brief observation.

The small amount of emotional attention and the intellectual paucity in the homes in which the children live almost from birth onwards, were not taken into account in the test situation and in the evaluation of the children.

This situation, which contravenes human rights, was denounced even by the people's deputies of the St. Petersburg city council during the Second International Conference on Human Rights in 1990 in St. Petersburg. In these children's homes, according the peoples deputies, the children receive an inadequate education and often no education at all.

Many parents have reported they were obliged to place their handicapped children in these state homes and not to tell other persons that they were parents of a mentally handicapped child. Thus, according to their statements, it was not permitted to talk to other people about the problem of mental handicap.

There were and there still are only two possibilities for most mentally handicapped children:

- Either they live in a closed institution under so-called state education and the conditions prevalent there such as isolation, generally inadequate care, and training which is limited mostly to self-sufficiency and to productive usefulness;
- Or they stay with their parents, as often was and still is the case in village communities.

In the official Soviet view the family was not seen as the natural environment into which the mentally handicapped child should be incorporated. Parents were considered to be incompetent on the subject. This is associated with the Communist theory of the development of secondary defects. Living together with non-trained persons is expected to produce 'social deformity'. Thus there will be a risk that inappropriate behavior will occur, that the handicap will not be compensated for but exacerbated.

For this reason families are given neither professional counseling nor support by special services.

There is also no training for social workers. As a result many families with handicapped children in the countries of the Eastern bloc are often reliant on self-support and on help from their extended families. Handicapped children and adults, who live with their families, generally receive no medical and educational aids and are, in practice, ignored.

Families who have a handicapped child also do not have a right to a larger apartment. There are practically no day centers. For handicapped children, mothers who keep their children at home cannot go to work, which means that the financial situation of their families is increasingly strained.

In many cases the fathers simply leave their family, as they cannot, or do not want to, bear the whole responsibility for the family situation.

Neighborhoods often discriminate against families with handicapped children as well. The non-handicapped children in the family suffer as a result and the psychological burdens on members of the family are intensified. If the rejection of handicapped children in the neighborhood is very severe they may live in isolation in their parent's house and have contact only with the family.

In the boarding schools for retarded children there are some therapies such as motor therapy, speech therapy, music therapy or occupational training. However the curriculum is very limited and is oriented towards practical skills, particularly towards those which produce useful products. There is, in practice, no training for weaker children, as they are considered to be incapable of learning. So-called profoundly handicapped children, who, in the West, go to schools for children with a mental handicap, are completely excluded from any form of organized training.

In one children's home visited in Moscow, about twenty profoundly handicapped children were looked after by one person who had no professional training. These children never see the ones in the neighboring beds, they are never taken out into the yard, they never see the sky, only the white ceiling over their beds.

In another children's home in Moscow, as in other institutions, many bed-ridden children lie crowded, bed by bed, in often evil-smelling rooms. Generally one non-trained person is in charge of fifteen to twenty such children, one nurse is available for eighty of them. The children are shaven to protect against lice, and poorly dressed. They often slide about on the floor without toys or push each other about. Children who are victims of social neglect may be put into groups with retarded and mentally handicapped children, where there may also be children with physical handicaps, such as cerebral palsy, children with behavior problems, and even normal children, who somehow found their way into these homes.

Not infrequently, individual children or whole groups are sent from 'normal' children's homes to those for the handicapped, if, during the annual check-up, lack of nutrition and poor care is discovered.

As mental handicap is seen to be a disease, medical care is available in the institutions. Thus children from normal children's homes can also profit from it.

The catastrophic economic situation in eastern Europe, which makes improvements in the social sector almost impossible, means that problems in the field of support for the disabled can only be attempted with very great efforts and can only be implemented over a long period of time.

This part of Europe is desperately seeking support and professional know-how from the West. Only in this way will inroads be made on the devastating consequences of a policy which was directed against the lives of handicapped persons.

Finally I should like to include here the report of a social worker who visited a home for children said to be incapable of learning near Minsk in Belarus in 1994.

VISIT TO A HOME FOR INEDUCABLE CHILDREN IN NOWINKI NEAR MINSK, 1994

The penetrating smell of a chlorinated disinfectant hangs in the air. When I see the metal bars in front of the door to the department for the 'severely handicapped' I know that I am in for a horrifying sight.

The barred door is opened and then the other door. We gaze into a dark, unlit corridor, from which an indescribable smell emanates. Behind the door lies a bundle, which at first is not recognizable as a human being. His torso has been tightly bound up with sheets, a helpless measure by the staff to prevent him injuring himself and others.

We go further and come to a day room in which about ten children and young persons are lying on the floor. Half of them are tied up with sheets in the manner described above. They wear either torn clothing or no clothing at all. They rock back and forth, utter cries or move their heads suddenly from one side to another. All of them have shaved heads. Two elderly women in white overalls are sitting on a bench, the only piece of furniture in the room. They are the only staff in a ward with thirty severely handicapped children.

In another room there are thirty beds in rows of four. They are clean, newly made-up and the bedclothes have amusing patterns. There is sun-light streaming into the room. I am told that the children do not use this room and these beds. When I ask why, the head of the institution tells me that they are too handicapped to lie in beds. For this reason they sleep on the concrete floor of the day room.

The manager tells me that many visitors from the West had already been there and had promised help, but that none had come. When I ask him about the bales of children's clothing filling up half of his office, he tells me that all these children do with their clothing is tear it up and for this reason he cannot do much with this sort of assistance. What is necessary is renovation, individual attention to the children, and the installation of trained staff. I decide not to take any photos, in order not to humiliate the children and the staff still further.

Behind another door there is another day-room. Here, too, the sight of bald children's heads and naked bodies wound up in sheets. There are various kinds of handicap, such as microcephalus or hydrocephalus. The volunteer who made it possible for me to visit the homes tells me that students of 'defectology' regularly visit this group to observe the various clinical manifestations of 'mental handicap' themselves.

On the journey back I confront the representative of the local social authority with the demands of the UN Children's Convention, which has been signed by the Republic of Belarus, and which states that a mentally or physically handicapped child should lead a fulfilled and humane life under conditions which guarantee the dignity of the child, promote his independence and facilitate his active participation in the life of society.

The woman is near to tears, as she herself considers conditions in the home to be degrading. But she has no means of solution as there is a lack of finances and of trained personnel.

Concluding Remarks

In many countries in the world, not least because of international cooperation, there has been considerable progress in the efforts to gain improvements in the situation of mentally handicapped persons and their families. However, on some parts of our earth, innumerable mentally handicapped persons and their families still suffer a wretched existence because of the socioeconomic, political or other circumstances which exist where they live.

The organizations for persons with a mental handicap in the privileged parts of our world are especially called upon to make their contribution to putting an end to this intolerable situation!

SECTION IV

Self-Advocacy Issues

15

On Being Left Out

Barb Goode
British Columbia, Canada

It was CACL's self-advocate "Advisory Committee" that had permission from the Supreme Court to appear before it and to be heard in the *Eve* case. It was our opinion about sterilization that the Supreme Court agreed with. But the newspaper and television reporters didn't want to interview us. They were not interested in our opinions. They only wanted to interview people who were not labeled to hear their opinions about sterilization.

It is not only society that shuts out people with labels. The same thing can happen inside families. Often, parents and other family members do not expect people with a disability to have anything important to say, even when it is about their own lives and well being. Very often, they are not even included in family discussions about their financial future, like when families discuss their wills and their plans for the future with the brothers and sisters who don't have disabilities but not with the ones who do.

People in the Association who are family members need to think very carefully about this. We can't expect society to recognize the equality of people with disabilities if we, in the Association, don't always recognize it ourselves.

Self-advocates for Equality are looking at the *Terry Urquhart* and *Latimer* cases and [are] considering how best to make politicians and other influential people more aware of the attitudes and prejudices that put people with disabilities at a disadvantage. We have asked other interested people to work with us in this effort because it is not a disability problem. It is a community problem. No one has the right to say

---

Editor's note: In the 1970s a Self-Advocate Advisory Committee (SAAC) was established by the Canadian Association for Community Living (CACL). Its purpose was to ensure that members of the CACL Board were aware at all times of the issues considered most relevant by people who had been labeled as having an intellectual disability. The right of people not to be sterilized without personal consent was one of those issues. Barb Goode of British Columbia, a former Chairperson of the Committee, led the move for intervention in the Supreme Court hearing on the Eve case.

Barb Goode was the first self-advocate on the CACL Board of Directors. She also served as the first Chairperson of Inclusion International's Self-Advocacy Committee.

that my life is less valuable that yours or that your life is less valuable than someone else's.

Often, a person with a disability wants to learn about an issue and would be able to understand it, but the language in which it is written or in which it is discussed it too complicated. When it is full of words that only certain people would understand, it leaves the person out. The person is then denied the opportunity to learn and to understand the issue. That handicaps the person. This is a problem for many people. Not just [for] people with certain labels.

Plain language is a kind of "ramp" that we have to build to give people access to understanding things. Although there have been some improvements, we have to build a lot more plain language ramps to make sure we don't leave people out.

Perhaps we also have to build ramps to help other people to know how to listen to us and how to believe that everyone has something worthwhile to say and something of value to give to society.

16

Gentle Words To Self-Advocate Friends

Robert Perske
Darien, CT

I'm a very lucky man
This is the third time I've had a chance to speak to you.
I love doing it.

I got to know some of you during the hearings on the Pennhurst institution.
I remember when you started to speak for yourselves.
    It was rough.
    It was hard.
    It was scary.

But do you know what?
    The more you spoke for yourselves
    — it got easier.
    — you did better.

But do you remember what it was like before you started speaking for yourselves?
    I do.
    I worked in an institution.
    And we institutional workers were in control.
    How did we do it?

    We told everybody that you couldn't speak for yourselves. "Only we can speak for you," we said.
    We refused to see you as individuals. "John, I know you'd love walking in town, but if we let you go, we'd have to let everyone go," we said.

Editor's Note: For a number of years, the author of this statement enjoyed a close relationship with the members of Speaking for Ourselves, in Pennsylvania. Then came an occasion to reflect on their good work.

We herded you like sheep. We said things like, "Okay folks. Head 'em up. Let's move out." It's time to go to the dining hall ... or it's time to head for the showers ... or it's time to go to bed."

We did the choosing for you. "What's that, John? You don't want to take a shower? Okay, you have a choice to make: One: You can take a shower. Or two: You can go to the seclusion room. It's your choice." (Some choice!)

We forced you to look good. During the Saturday night dances at the institution where I once worked, we, the staff members, moved across the dance floor toward couples who were dancing too close. "Joe and Sally," we would smile and say in a soft voice, "you are dancing too close. This is Number One." (Everyone knew that if they received a smile and a Number Three, they would be restricted from the dances for six months.)

We kept you from being heroes. I recall how staff members of the institute where I worked were called one night to the institution to search for a resident who had wondered off the grounds and into the woods. Two teenage residents asked me it they could help search for their friend. I asked the superintendent. He said if was okay if they stayed with me. The two residents found their lost friend! After all, they hiked and camped in the woods during supervised recreation programs all the time. They knew the woods better than we did.

So we tried to control you.
    We thought we were doing it for your own good.
    We didn't know any better.
    Then *you* started speaking for yourselves.
    You got better and better at it.

And do you know what?
    You proved us wrong.
    Just look at what you have done:

Jerome Ianuzzi and Carol Talley got married and so did Frank Wetmore and Mary Ella White. Do you think you could have gotten married when we spoke for you? Now all we can say is, "Congratulations, Mr. and Mrs. Ianuzzi," and "Congratulations, Mr. and Mrs. Wetmore."

DeWeese White spoke for himself. He walked out of the sheltered workshop. He got himself a job as a front-of-the-store "greeter" at K-Mart. He welcomes people and directs them to the proper sections of the store.

Richard Humer left his home to live with two close friends.

Roland Johnson made a presentation to President Bush. It was even shown on national television. Could you have done this if you had never started to speak for yourself?

Fifteen of you now go to college. You have been paired off with other college students, and you go to classes together.

Jerry Ellis and Lester Noch, you've been friends ever since your days together at the Pennhurst Center. Now you live together in your own house. And you picked that house.

George Ware just went out and got his own job. Such nerve. He'd never been trained in vocational rehab!

Many of you worked on the project that helped the National Park Service shape up their presentations and attitudes at Independence Hall. You taught them about "barriers" ... about treating people as human beings ... about where to stand ... and what to say.

Debbie Robinson, you helped try to save Robert Wayne Sawyer from execution. You got your brothers and sisters to send letters to Governor Edwards of Louisiana.

You testify before legislatures, governors, presidents and town councils. You always seem to be testifying. And do you know what? These officials often listen to you better than they do the rest of us!

Your new mission statement is beautiful! Just look at what you are saying:

> "We seek to be an independent community organization controlled by people with disabilities who help us:
> 1. Find a voice for ourselves. (That's great!)
> 2. Teach the public about the needs and wishes and potential of people with disabilities. (That's beautiful!)
> 3. Speak out on important issues. (Keep doing it!)
> 4. Support each other through sharing, leadership development, and helping and encouraging each other." (I love it!)

Even so, why not consider a fifth point—one that gets you looking outside your circle?
Proposed #5. Support each other to be good givers in the neighborhood.
Why? Because you are becoming strong.
And a wise leader named Gandhi once said "Only the strong can be truly kind."
Think about that.
Then, with your newfound strength, think about ...
SHOWING LOVE TO YOUR NEIGHBORS.
    Some will be grateful.
    But some won't.
    Love them anyway!
DOING GOOD THINGS TO OTHERS.
    Some will thank you.
    But some won't.
    Do good anyway!

BEING KIND TO UNDERDOGS.
    Some will be better for it.
    But some will not.
    Be kind to underdogs anyway!

People like you can make a good neighborhood better. And do you know what? Some neighborhoods will not be as lucky as yours. Because there's not enough people like you to go around. And some neighborhoods will have to do without.

I wish you well.

17

Who Teaches Us?

Michael J. Kennedy*
Center for Human Policy, Syracuse University

In this piece, I want to discuss my personal development as a self-advocate and as a person who speaks about self-advocacy around the country. I feel that my development has gone along parallel with the growth of the self-advocacy movement, so I will also refer a little bit to the history of the movement. In doing both of these, I must talk about Gunnar and Rosemary Dybwad. They have both done so much to promote self-advocacy and to make sure that whatever they did they always included people with disabilities. They heard our points of view no matter what the issue and supported our self-advocacy movement,

    I want to start by talking about what self-advocacy is and what it means to us to be heard in this way. For years, we were told that people with disabilities don't know what they want or need, and that we didn't have thoughts and opinions worth listening to. To have people like Gunnar and Rosemary open the door and listen carefully to what we have to say has meant a great deal to me personally and the movement. They helped to pave the way so that we could feel free to say what we wanted. It can be really scary to go up against a system that thinks it knows better than you what you need. When people that are important within the system listen to us, that fear is bearable. Now, I feel I have been given the opportunity to tell the system what I think about how services are delivered. I can play an active role in the way my own services are provided, and I can also speak out on issues involving other people and help them feel more comfortable in speaking out on their own behalf. It is a

---

The preparation of this article was supported by the Center on Human Policy, School of Education. Syracuse University, through a subcontract with the Research and Training Center on Community Living, University of Minnesota, supported by the U.S. Department of Education, Office of Special Education and Rehabilitative Services, National Institute on Disability and Rehabilitation Research (NIDRR), through Contract No. Hl33B980047. Members of the Center are encouraged to express their opinions. However, these do not necessarily represent the official position of NIDRR and no endorsement should be inferred.

---

* Assisted by Bonnie Shoultz.

great feeling to know that I and so many other people can express ourselves now, and that we will be heard.

My first contact with Gunnar and Rosemary was in 1984. When I was 23 years old, I was hired by the Center on Human Policy as a Self-Advocacy coordinator, only a year or so after I came out of the Syracuse Developmental Center (SDC). The other coordinator was Pat Killius, a woman who had also been a resident of SDC. Our funding came from the J. Stewart Mott Foundation and its purpose was to make links between the self-advocacy and independent joining movements. This was my first job. A graduate student, Deborah Olson, who is now a professor at the University of Oregon, supported us. In 1984, People First of Washington held a five-day international meeting in Tacoma, WA. People came from many countries, including Canada, England, New Zealand, Australia, and the U.S. Rosemary Dybwad came and participated in the whole meeting. Her being there made me feel respected and really good. Seeing that someone that famous believed in us made me feel like my voice was equally important to hers. She told us that our voices were just as significant as hers, regardless of our disabilities. From then on I had a new sense of strength or belonging. I was confirmed in my feeling that this line of work was meant for me and was where I belonged.

Shortly after Tacoma, I met Gunnar. Gunnar was then on the Syracuse University faculty, and one day he came to one of the Center's staff meetings. Even though he lived in Boston and was on the Brandeis University faculty, he used to fly to Syracuse one day a week to teach his course. He shared some stories about people he had met when he visited institutions during his travels, about how the residents were shoved on back wards and about how he helped some people get out of institutions, He emphasized that we are people, not just a disability. That told me that, like Rosemary, he believed in us as people who could contribute to our communities and our society if given the right opportunities.

Before that, I knew I had a voice but I wondered whether it was a voice that anyone could hear. Was I speaking just to get things off my chest, or was I speaking to make changes in the world? Once I knew that what I said would be heard by important people, I realized that I needed to learn about how the system worked. If I didn't know that, I wouldn't be effective enough to help other people know what their rights were and how to exercise them. I asked questions of some of the people I was closest to. I went to meetings and conferences, and I used the resources of the Center on Human Policy. Deborah Olson was a great resource for Pat and me. She suggested ways I could get answers to my questions, and she arranged meetings for us with people like Steve Taylor, the Center on Human Policy director. We looked up the writings of Burton Blatt and books about self-advocacy and independent living. Debbie read these to us, since neither of us could read.

We spent a couple of weeks where we went through different things to see! What would work for each of us. For example, she didn't know that I had trouble reading, so at first she would write things out for me and have me try to read them back to her. I could read some but not all the words in a sentence, and that told her that I needed to have other ways of learning. Then she thought of putting information on tapes that I could listen to. Pat is blind and cannot use Braille, so the tapes worked for her as well.

So we would be more effective in our speaking, Debbie helped us practice. We did role-playing, and she made symbols for me to help me keep track of what I was planning to say. Sometimes she would take photographs that we would make into a slide show for me. The symbols and slides did not help Pat because she couldn't see them, so Debbie found other ways to work with her. Since I am an auditory learner some of those worked with me as well. The tapes were great—they might be about the basic ideas behind self-advocacy and the People First movement, for example.

We were expected, when we gave a talk, to be accurate about these things. We could not just talk off the tops of our heads. Self-advocacy doesn't mean that people should automatically believe you just because you have a disability. It puts a lot of responsibility on the self-advocate to know what he or she is talking about. Debbie used to say that we needed to be accurate because someone in the audience might ask questions that we couldn't answer, or they might take action on what we said. It is a bit scary to be in this position, because you hope that what you try to teach is instilling the right things in your audience. You want them to develop confidence in themselves and to act on what they believe, but you don't want them to go away believing things that aren't true.

Here is an example: you don't want people to think having rights means that just because they have a disability they don't have responsibilities and can do anything they want to do. One person at a conference in the Midwest said, "I want my rights as a self-advocate, but I don't think I should have to take responsibility for anything." In his case, he just wanted his agency to accept and carry out his rights, but he didn't want to be a part of making sure that it happened. My answer to him was that in order for the self-advocate to have his rights, he has to take responsibility for himself, and if he's not willing to do that, he can't complain if his agency makes decisions for him. Before I started learning how to give talks, I wouldn't have known how to formulate an answer like that. What Debbie and others at the Center helped me do was to think through issues like that.

Since those days, I have gained even more exposure to self-advocacy and have learned more ways to help other people with disabilities who have had less experience than I have had. I know that others can learn just the way that I did, and can develop confidence in themselves, if they have the support and tools they need. I have watched the self-advocacy movement grow. When I started, it was already pretty strong, but there were only a few state organizations, and there were none in the Northeast except for Speaking for Ourselves in Pennsylvania. Now there are something like 40 state organizations and hundreds of local groups. When I give presentations it seems like everyone is familiar with self-advocacy and wants to know more about it. In the early days, many of the people I talked to hadn't even beard about it.

The ties between the self-advocacy movement, which is made up mostly of people with developmental disabilities, and the independent living movement, which was historically founded by people with physical disabilities, are strengthening all the time. Our self-advocacy leaders, those who are on the board of directors of the national organization, Self-Advocates Becoming Empowered, are learning how to be effective at the national level, and that is really exciting. I feel I have lived through some challenging times, and things have happened that I could never have predicted. Self-advocacy has become a movement that has strength and influence.

I always tell people, though, that I don't want self-advocacy to become just another buzz word that agencies use to try to look good. I want it to be a living experience, not just something on paper, and I tell them that. Now it is common for important people to say they are listening to our ideas and I believe that many of them really are listening. We still have those who say "Yeah, we hear you," but who don't do anything to change things. That is why we still need a self-advocacy movement. One person speaking out can't do as much to influence people to change as a whole group can. Numbers really do make a difference. But along with that, it has been incredibly important to have important people as our allies. We can't pretend that important people don't matter. They often have power that we haven't had, and they need to be willing to share the power with us. We need them to influence the people around them to listen and work to share their power with us as well,

I don't mean to say that we who have disabilities are not important people. I believe that we are important now and are becoming more powerful and important all the time. We are learning more about our own power and how to use it all the time, thanks to the movement that we have created. It was wonderful at the beginning to learn about our potential by having people like Rosemary and Gunnar listen to us. I hope that future generations will feel that we, the ones who speak out today, are listening to them and helping them see our potential. We are the important people they will learn from.

18

Tokenism—It Doesn't Look Good!!!

Liz Obermayer
Department of Mental Retardation, Commonwealth of Massachusetts

BEING A BOARD MEMBER, NOT A TOKEN

I am a self-advocate, and one of the most important things I do is to work on boards of directors. It is a glory to be on a board, it is fun, but we need to question things. Self-advocates can not just **be on** the board but we need to **be a part of** the board. There is a big difference between being a valued board member, and being just a token. It is a big honor, but it is a big responsibility too. You need to be able to contribute. I know from personal experience.

When I first began to be a board member, I was caught up in the glory and was proud and honored to be on the board. I got to see all the important notes and to hear a lot of important information.

It is really hard for a self-advocate who is just learning to be a self-advocate to understand what tokenism is all about. A few years ago, I was on a board that oversaw the services that I received in New Jersey, and I felt very honored to be there at first. Then I felt like they were not listening to me and all they wanted from me was to say that they had a person with a disability on the board. I made suggestions to the board based on what I was hearing my friends who also received services were saying and I was feeling. I was feeling like the board was hearing me with only "one ear," meaning they were not hearing me at all. I finally "woke up" and left the board. I realized that the board members were not respecting what I had to offer, **they were just half listening to me. Boards need to use the person for their abilities, not their disabilities.** I finally figured out they were treating me like a token only seeing my disabilities. I thought I should quit. So I did! I told them as much as I could about why I was quitting, but I do not know if they truly understood why I quit. But if they did not understand, it is not my fault.

TOKENISM DOESN'T LOOK GOOD FOR A LOT OF REASONS

When you treat someone like a token, it makes the person feel like you really don't appreciate them for what they can offer. It makes them feel like you only see their disabilities and worry about what they can't do. People get tired of only being seen as having disabilities. They don't like talking about their disabilities all the time. They would rather show people their abilities, show what they **can** do.

WAYS TO STOP TOKENISM

First, involve people with disabilities on boards of directors. If you choose not to include people with disabilities on your board, then you are taking a risk for people to say that you are not an inclusive group. You are missing a "link" or a voice that is very important. The people who benefit from your services really know better than you how to improve your services or what's good about them. People with disabilities's voices are probably the most important ones around the table. You will include parents and family members on the boards to hear their perspectives on issues, then why can't you include people with disabilities?

Second, involve more than one self-advocate. Agencies shouldn't use just one person for a lot of committees or projects—they might get burnt out. There are a lot of good self-advocates who want to be on boards. Different people have different interests. Let the person decide for themselves what they want to be involved with; it might not be the same as what you want them be involved with. The reason why two people are good is because one person might feel like he or she can't speak up. They might not feel comfortable speaking up without a friend who know what they are going through with having a disability. The other reason it that is could also make the person feel like a "token".

Third, support true participation. People need support. At meetings, people need support to participate. For example, if the board is talking about the finances—then it is your responsibility to help the person understand the information (if that is needed) as long as it takes to do that. Don't just say "they don't understand". Help them. For that matter, this should include any and all information. This rule goes both ways—the person needs to take some responsibility for speaking up and asking you, as the support person, for help and you should do the same.

The support person should sit beside the person that you're supporting. If you want to sit by your friend or need to sit by someone else for a reason, then the person you are supporting won't feel like they can ask you questions if needed. Ask if that's what they want. They might want to have the support done during breaks, lunch or after the meeting (set up a different time)

When I started with the TASH board, in the beginning I used a lot of staff time for support. Now that I am feeling comfortable, I still lean on staff to explain things to me before and after meetings, but in meetings I like to depend on the board members who are my friends for support during a meeting. Between meetings, if I have a question, I will ask staff to explain something to me.

A Good Support Person and a Bad One

You might think there's nothing to think about when you agree to be a support person for someone with a disability, but there are some things to think about if want to be a good and successful one.

First—get to know the person—that might include going out for breakfast, lunch or dinner. If that is not affordable, then just meet and get to know and feel comfortable with each other. It's just as important for you to feel comfortable with the person you are supporting as it is for them to feel comfortable with you. From my past experience, if the person doesn't feel like they can trust or even feel comfortable with you, then they won't get something out of the meeting because the person might not even ask questions of you if they don't understand. They could look out of the window and not pay attention to what is being discussed, and not participate in the meeting.

If you are inviting someone with a disability to be on the board, then you should be ready to listen to the person, even if the person is going to say something that you don't necessarily agree with. For example, if the person is unhappy with the services he or she is getting from your agency, they might want to talk about that. This might be hard for you to listen to, but you ask for their opinions. It is your responsibility to listen, after all, they do receive services or could benefit from your services.

The support person who you assign to the person should be available to go over the board materials with the person with a disability before and after the meeting. The support person should be a member of the board or committee. It is easy for the board to pass that responsibility on to an advisor or a friend of the person with a disability or the staff, but then the person with a disability might feel like they are different than any one else. The other reason for this is because the person who is helping the board member with a disability will not know what's going on at the meeting because he or she don't go to the meetings, and they should!

Before you invite someone with a disability to be on the board, you or your board really should think about why the board wants to do this. It can be a wonderful experience for you, the person, but only if it is done in the right and thoughtful way.

Do not invite people to be on the board just because the State is telling you to. Do this because you think inviting people with disabilities is the right thing to do and you want to hear from these people!!

19

Who Speaks for Whom?
Issues of Advocacy

Ann Shearer & Alison Wertheimer
London, England

In 1971, a small group of concerned British citizens launched Campaign for the Mentally Handicapped. It quickly became known simply as CMH, which was not just punchier for publicity purposes but a useful cover for increasing internal debate: mentally handicapped people? campaign with? By the start of the 1980s, the official name was 'CMH: The Campaign for Mentally Handicapped People'. Nowadays, it is called 'Values into Action (VIA)', and the small print adds that it is 'the national campaign with people who have learning difficulties'. The changes of title reflect a huge change in perception over the past 30 years among service planners and providers no less than many people with learning difficulties themselves. Yet the questions remain: who can legitimately speak with and for whom in the complexities of our social organizations? What are the implications for deeper social cohesion or fragmentation of our provisional and evolving answers? In this at least, people with learning difficulties have equal share in some of the most pressing issues of our time.

When CMH began, it was a very new sort of organization in its field. For whom was it claiming to speak and what was its legitimacy? In those days, it was generally assumed that the interests of people with learning difficulties were probably coincident with those of their parents and certainly most properly represented by them, sometimes in uneasy alliance with their medical and other professional advisors. CMH numbered parents among its activists but it was not — unlike the giants in the field, the Spastics Society and National Association for Mentally Handicapped Children (MENCAP) — a parent-led organization. Some of CMH's members were pro-

---

Ann Shearer was a co-founder of CMH and worked with it for fifteen years alongside her career as a journalist, lecturer and international consultant on services for people with, learning difficulties. She is now a Jungian analyst in private practice in London.

Alison Wertheimer was Director of CMH (now Values Into Action) from 1980 to 1987. Since then, she has worked as a freelance researcher and writer, with a continuing focus on people with learning difficulties. She now also works as a counselor and trainer.

fessionals, too, but it did not claim to represent their interests either. Who were these people? As one of us (AS) well remembers, the antagonism towards CMH from established groupings was fierce and often painful. It is in no small measure thanks to the support of James Loring, the then director of the Spastics Society, and especially of Rosemary and Gunnar Dybwad, who brought an international perspective and hugely generous network of experience from the start, that VIA exists today.

Yet CMH had its own legitimacy too, and it was of a contemporary sort. The widespread challenge to established authority that grew internationally during the 1960s had touched Britain's welfare state as well. An increasing number of small pressure groups criticised the ever-more evident inadequacies of the system and produced their own plans for reform. Characteristically, these were not organizations of involved professionals or service-receivers. They took their legitimacy from the fact that their members, as concerned citizens and taxpayers, claimed every right – and indeed duty to speak out. In so far as CMH had a model, it was the Child Poverty Action Group, whose founding members were neither children nor poor, but respected academics whose relentless critique of social policy became an indispensable feature of public debate.

So from the start, CMH was in one sense at least a 'mainstream' organization, just as it was dedicated to campaigning for mainstream opportunities for people with learning difficulties. Importantly, the form of the organization and the content of its message went together, just as the form of the older 'special interest' organizations went with their own more segregationist policies. From the very start, CMH's main message was that the large mental handicap hospitals should be closed. This was an essentially moral message, and its very simplicity, unclouded by political or professional concerns, together with the energy and enthusiasm with which it was preached, gave it a particular impact.

What CMH could not do, in those heady early days, was to claim that it spoke for or with anyone except its own members and others who shared its inclusive social vision. Yet only a year after it began, I was already addressing this issue with the first of a series of residential conferences or 'participation events' that strengthened its claim to speak on behalf of people with learning difficulties. The inspiration for these events came from a Swedish report of the first recorded discussion of services among people with learning difficulties. In its series of conferences, CMH went further, by bringing together delegates who lived in hospitals and hostels, or used other service, with delegates who provided such services. These events, with their mixture of discussion and other shared activities, were often intensely moving and even painful, both for those who spoke of a lifetime of limitation and for staff who experienced, however briefly, a radical new equality between themselves and those they 'cared for' (Shearer, 1972,1973; CMH,1973). The format was ground-breaking and became internationally influential. The events themselves become seen as 'Powerful British examples of how mentally handicapped people [sic] can be given a voice of their own' (Williams and Shoultz, 1982:166).

What happened to those voices of the early '70s? Certainly CMH was able to draw on them to strengthen its own moral authority in meetings with government ministers and professional leaders and to dramatize its own arguments for reform. The mingling of policy analysis with personal statements from those who had to live with the consequences of policy decisions became a hallmark of CMH publications, and in this it again reflected a 'mainstream': 'the personal is the political' as the contemporary feminist slogan influentially declared. As director of CMH at this period, one of us (AW) recalls how our evidence to a Parliamentary Select Committee on community care really made an impact when we not only offered policy-related proposals but told MPs about individual people with learning difficulties, and the changes that a move from hospital to community had made to their lives (Wertheimer, 1984).

While CMH could draw on the voices of people with learning difficulties to strengthen its own campaigning stance, there was little evidence of those voices exercising a direct influence on local or national decision-making. Nevertheless, they were beginning to be heard through the growing number of 'user' or 'student' committees set up in adult day facilities, which sometimes achieved modest changes within their establishments. The foundations were being laid for what was to become a UK self-advocacy movement in the 1980s.

That movement led self-advocacy out of service systems and into a more independent — and even international — environment. Once again, CMH could claim a part in preparing the ground for this. In 1979, one of its founder members, Paul Williams, and Alan Salmon, a young man with learning difficulties (the son of another member) visited the United States on a Rosemary Dybwad Fellowship to learn about its self-advocacy movement and bring its experience back to Britain (Williams and Shoultz, 1982). Three years later, the London Division of MENCAP which nationally remained a parent-focused organization, set up a Participation Forum. It also joined forces with CMH to cosponsor the First International Self-Advocacy Conference, held, in Washington State in August 1984.

That event was a turning point. Delegates returned to Britain inspired by the example of their American friends and determined to set up their own organization. By the end of the year, delegates had formed People First of London and Thames. Four years later, this organization hosted the second International Self-Advocacy Conference in London. As the movement grew, so did the role of the organizations which it had long spoken for and with perceptibly changed. CMH became a member of a Supporters' Group which produced the first British training materials for self-advocacy (CMH, 1984).

As People First quickly discovered, the demands on this fledgling organization were enormous. Members were under considerable pressure, with requests flooding in for self-advocates to speak at conferences, run training events and help new groups to start up around Britain. Self-advocacy, it seemed, was an idea whose time had come. It was also, throughout the '80s and well into the '90s, an idea that was caught up in a far wider political mainstream, and this has brought both opportunities and difficulties.

At the start of the 1980s, a Conservative government had recently embarked on what was to become nearly two decades in office. With a Prime Minister who roundly declared 'there is no such thing as community' and public health and welfare budget at a standstill or facing cutbacks, it soon became evident that the model for public services was now private enterprise, with those who used such services playing their part no longer as 'patients' or 'clients I put rather as 'customers' and 'consumers'. The radical implications of this philosophy for the British tradition of welfare provision are hard to overestimate (Shearer, 1991). The underlying post-war consensus of a 'common weal' was replaced by a philosophy of individual responsibility; a philosophy (if not a reality) of cooperation in the sharing of resources was replaced by the legitimation of competition.

In this fragmentation, service users have theoretically been given primacy. Newly empowered as 'consumers' or 'customers', they can call on Charters of Rights about everything from education to health services to railways. Yet too often the range of provision that would make 'consumer choice' a reality is simply lacking. The hollowness of much of the rhetoric of 'consumer empowerment has a deeper dimension too. There is little recognition of the simple fact that people mostly turn to health and social services not when they are powerful and fit, but when they are weak and in need of support and care. In the rejection of both the paternalistic model of 'speaking for' and the cooperative one of 'speaking with', in favor of 'speak for yourself', governments may reckon to save money through a fantasy of a welfare constituency made up of strong, independent and always-adequate 'customers'. But in the real world, individuals with sickness and groups which are vulnerable, may suffer.

As users of health, social and educational services, people with learning difficulties are seen as part of this consumer movement, and both individuals and self-advocacy groups can take legitimation and strength from the philosophy as well as learning to live with its consequences. Community care policies emphasize choice and control, giving people a greater say in how they live their lives and the services they need to help them do so' (Secretaries of State, 1989, para.1.8). Yet as other individuals and groups are also discovering, the reality is all too often somewhat different. The language of the market place is attractive when the customer can choose between shops or stalls. But choice in welfare services can end up as Hobson's Choice: 'Hobson's day center... Hobson's residential care home' (Midwinter, 1990). Who will speak for and with people with learning difficulties in their pursuit of the services they need? As the philosophy and practice of self-advocacy becomes stronger, the question may become more not less complicated. In recent years, for instance, MENCAP has become a much more actively campaigning organization and now claims to bring its considerable influence to speak on behalf of people with learning difficulties. Yet it is not so long since it was strongly attacked by People

First for maintaining its 'Little Stephen' logo, the image of a pitiful little boy, which did nothing at all to empower people with learning difficulties but a great deal, apparently, to raise funds. People First – and the changing times too – made their point. Little Stephen finally died in 1992, when MENCAP started to use photographs of real individuals with learning difficulties to support its emphasis on opportunities for 'Making the Most of Life'. But the relatively recent debate over Little Stephen illustrates how great a perceptual gulf may separate even those who are ostensibly on the same side.

Even when perceptions are apparently shared, questions remain. People First has had to try to strike a difficult balance between getting the support it needs and protecting itself from being taken over by professionals. At the same time, it has not been easy for it to find other allies. One of the strengths and of self-advocacy in the US, from a British perspective, has been the growth of coalitions of people with different disabilities, seeking common cause. In Britain in the 1970s, CMH was an active member of the Disability Alliance – a coalition of organizations which spoke for and sometimes with different groups of people with disabilities. In the 1980s, links were established between People First and some other organisations, notably the British Council of Disabled People. But on the whole it has been hard for people with learning difficulties to make common cause with other disabled citizens.

The reasons for this seem complex. People with learning difficulties may need to feel confident about putting forward their own views before they feel ready to join with others; some people with physical or sensory impairments may be reluctant to be associated with those with learning difficulties. What seems sure is that in the culture of competition, rather than cooperation, that has characterized Britain for nearly two decades, it has been harder rather than easier to form alliances. And in turn, of course, that may make it more difficult for any of the disparate groups to get the services they could perhaps jointly use, as harassed providers fall back on a policy of divide and rule.

With the election of the Labor government in 1997, Britain has begun to see some potentially significant shifts in the way society views itself, the values it espouses and the mechanisms which enable people to participate in decision-making. This government promises to work towards the creation of an inclusive society, one which recognizes, values and celebrates diversity and difference and draws in those individuals and groups who have hitherto been marginalized or excluded.

The force of the rhetoric has yet to be matched by action, and for both advocates and self-advocates, the challenge remains: how can people with learning difficulties become part of the promised inclusive society? Certainly those who want to make their collective views known continue to face many obstacles to legitimate participation. It can often remain true that self-advocacy is in danger of becoming 'no more than a fashion accessory for fashion conscious services' (Dowson, 1990:2). Those who are articulate may still be dismissed as 'not really handicapped'. Their claim to a representative voice may still be challenged. Their presence may still be merely a token as the meeting rubber-stamps what has already been decided elsewhere.

Yet people with learning difficulties are far from alone in experiencing such struggles. This is what the mainstream of social debate and negotiation is like and these are some of the fruits of inclusion in it. And there is good news too. People with learning difficulties are participating in policy- and decision-making, often in partnership with others. They are sharing conference platforms, undertaking joint training sessions, participating in service evaluation and sitting on boards of voluntary agencies alongside managers, politicians, professionals and parents.

Could such developments be seen as a new kind of shared participation, in which both people with learning difficulties and those who seek to speak with them are beginning to find a new cooperation that goes beyond the recent polarities? As important, are we beginning to see the growth of a participation in which both collective and individual views and voices have their own legitimacy? Are we witnessing an historical synchronicity in which the emergence of the self-advocacy movement among people with learning difficulties is paralleled by a dawning awareness of individual experiences and feelings? (Sinason, 1992). A new respect for both the collective and the individual experience is perhaps the next stage. As Rosemary Dybwad reminded delegates at the first International People First Conference in 1984, self-advocacy must grow at its own pace — that of those who are part of it. The same could as well be said for any movement which seeks to speak for and with people with learning difficulties and the individuals who make it what it is.

References

CMH. (1973). *A Workshop on Participation.* London: CMH.

CMH. (1984). *Learning About Self-Advocacy.* London: CMH.

Dowson, S. (1990).

Midwinter, E. (1990). 'Advise and Consent', in M. Bernard and F. Glendenning (eds.), *Advocacy, Consumerism and the Older Person.* Stoke on Trent: Beth Johnson Foundation.

Secretaries of State for Health, Social Security, Wales and Scotland. (1989). *Caring for people: Community care in the next decade and beyond.* London: Stationery Office.

Shearer, A. (1972). *Our Life.* London: CMH.

Shearer, A. (1973). *Listen.* London: CMH.

Shearer, A. (1991). *Who calls the shots? Public services and how they serve the people who use them.* London: King's Fund Centre.

Sinason, V. (1992). *Mental Handicap and the Human Condition. Approaches from the Tavistock.* London: Free Association Books.

Wertheimer, A. (1984). *Hope for the Future.* London: CMH.

Williams, P., and Shoultz, B. (1982). *We Can Speak for Ourselves.* Cambridge, MA: Brookline Books.

20

Not to Yield

Robert Williams Parsons Cutler, Jr.
Autism National Commitee

I, Robert Cutler, am 42 years old. I am autistic. I am proud to have this opportunity to present my experiences. I hope you see progression; but more importantly, happiness. Many know I have a dark side but I also have a bright side. I am now working on changing people's view of what I want.

My life has been hell because nobody truly understands autism. I live a life of hunting to survive. I enjoy the opportunity to choose who helps me. This was not always the case. Knowing how to type took 2 years of trial and error.

I am here because my family helped free me from Fernald to the point where I am a homeowner. Gunnar is a man whose words speak of love and hope. Gunnar supports my work. I am here as an example that if you give support and love to a human being who needs a hand up instead of pushing them down you will be amazed of the successes we can achieve. I want the world to positively support people with disabilities instead of housing us in institutions or group homes. I am angry that society still believes that pain and humiliation is the way to cure us or force us to act normal. I have autism. This is strange to you, but normal to me. Yes.

George, Sherri and my mom helped me get a home of my own. I thank them for believing that given a chance I could be part of the world. Mom fought the politicians with Rosemary and Gunnar to free me from Fernald. I have been through the group home phase to an apartment and finally my own home. Group homes control; workshops do too. I decide my life through typing called FC (Facilitated Communication) which I demonstrated at the Rosemary Ferguson Dybwad Memorial lecture at Brandeis University on November 12, 1998.

ABOUT MY DIFFICULTIES WITH AUTISM

Autism is a way of life. Until you stop trying to make us normal and work on acceptance and understanding about us individually, your attempts will be impossible. You need to find out how much of our disruptive behavior is because of allergy or neurological. Autism is not retardation.

Our daily life is full of rituals, just like normal people. But you study us because we are different. People with autism feel alienated because sometimes we want to be alone. They say "We are going into our world". But really we just need a break from life's challenges. Is asking our lives to be orderly and predictable any less than normal people want or any different?

I have stress just for being autistic. Your world depends on time. My world depends on sequence of events with no timeline. I belong in your world, but you will never understand my world. I need to understand stress.

I experience daily hatred and prejudices for one fact, I have Autism! It will be important to know that people with Autism are human beings. I am using past experience to make an honest assessment.

I was 8 months old when I started to read. My brain is too far advanced for a human being to grasp. My brain is hyper processing information ten times more than a regular brain.

I (sometimes) have difficulty in staying focused on task. It's like without a constant buildup of anxiety my body can't move. When I start breakfast it may take up to an hour just to cut the banana. When I am fast it's because I made my body feel anxious. Kinda tough way to live.

I get worried about body shaking. is permanent? I am hoping that my tremors are from stress and not seizures. Moving my body was difficult. Hands were shaking too. I voice the need to move more fluently. I don't know what is medicine and what is autistic. Lots of changes in my life. I never get used to change. It makes me powerless. I am edgy. I need more energy.

I hate seizures. They hurt my head. I want to be a good vice president (he is Vice President of the Autism National Committee and a Director of the Herb Lovett Memorial Fund). But I'm afraid seizures will destroy all my good qualities.

I feel useless when my body is stuck. It's like the body is frozen, but life keeps moving. I wish I could cope better. I am a man who does not want to be angry anymore. My life is hard. My body shakes. I feel tense and I don't know why. Until I can control my brain, I will need help. It is scary. Time will come when I will control my destiny. But for now, I can use everyone's input. It will benefit all.

ON SENSORY INTEGRATION

It helped my head feel better. It was hurting me. I need the walks. I needed to relax more. Summers (allergies) are hard on me. Can't wait till winter.

Life is not perfect. Let it be. Mystery is only a new challenge. I need to understand stress.

If you want, you can study me. You will probably end up with a library full of data, but you might get something more useful, a friendship with me. I am not the same as another person with Autism. I am me. We are all different. We need the people with Autism who speak to defend the voiceless person with Autism.

THE ROAD TO RECOVERY

In order to succeed
When others say you'll fail
Is to go into your boat
Put it in the ocean and set sail
To an uncharted world
Called confidence.

Once you have this
You can conquer the mysteries
Of the oceans wave
Going in and out
On the seashore in your brain.

It is easier to succeed
When others think you'll fail
The hard part is explaining to them
How simple it was to succeed
If only given a little more time
To have tried. Yes

When I am in heaven I will have autism. God just makes sure we all have a computer to FC.

About Facilitated Communication (FC)

If FC is fake then I'll tell you it's better than what behaviorists had tried on me. I type with the assistance from my friend of 12 years, Mark Powell.

Voices are not always good. Many people talk a lot but give useless information. We type to tell the truth. I feel pain in my head when I am asked to talk a lot. Often when many people are speaking, I hear static. I do better typing out my voice for people to hear. Typing will be a key for me to open up and share my knowledge and ideas. Knowledge is power you use to open minds of people stuck in old ideas. Try changing their minds. It would take a miracle.

I learned to believe in myself from typing words of Robert's mind on computers. It works! Knowing how to type took 2 years of trial and error. I can only type as much as my body allows me to do. It is hard but a little typing is better than none at all. I believe this is why others think FC fails, because some can only do a little while others can write books. FC is real. I look to a time when all people type.

It is a blessing that I am respected. But the ones who have no words deserve more respect.

Money and politics stop opportunities to communicate, Not enough cash and too much politics. We need to show the politicians that their programs can still make them money. Communication is our number one priority. If we communicated our needs there would be less behavior programs. No FC allowed throughout the system. They fear what we will say. HOPEFULLY, I can sway the politicians to allow a ten year trial and allow facilitated communication to happen. After ten years every child would have had the opportunity to speak.

It is important to help parents understand. Heaven knows, most parents feel ashamed, but God selected each for a reason. I will tell them to support FC and to never give up hope. Parents love your children; we love you. Maybe we can't talk but look into our soul. Yes.

Many people who try FC stop trying after a certain amount of time. But if they continued they would be typing now. Others put their children on hold waiting for the expert to come. We need to type, not wait. Every child needs a computer. I look to a time when all people with autism type. Give us the opportunity, we will not let you down. Doesn't matter how long it takes, but everyone should try and try again!

Typing is my voice. Typing is easier than words. Words are important, but writing lasts forever. Communication was scary when I first typed. A lot of fears about would I be listened to and emotional feelings about telling my family I loved them.

I might type alone someday. I dream of speaking clearly.

ABOUT MY FRIENDS AND FAMILY

I got opera young in Germany from my dad and mom. Music is the pulse of my life. I tried to be a good boy but autism started to take control of my mind and soul. I went down a path of destruction. For years I wandered through hell seeking value. I wish I could change the past, but I can't so I live in pain. I wanted to be a normal boy.

Just how far will a family go to help their son, brother, brother-in-law reach his dreams? I typed out dreams but all of you took up the challenge and made it a reality.

George, you are my brother and most of all my friend. Remember when we used to jump up and down on the beds. It would drive mom crazy, but do you think we can do it one more time? We are not too old. I was only joking, but it would be nice to go back like in the movie *Field of Dreams*.

Who came to my rescue when I was suffering with panic attacks? Answer, Mark, mom, George too. I love you all for your support and understanding. George, if something happens to mom or Mark, promise to protect me from evil.

Mom is the guiding force in my advocacy. Mom learned from Gunnar how to correct the injustice of Fernald. My mom spends hundreds of unpaid hours advocating for me, as well as other children. Mom, you have compassion for the disabled. When you are through with them they are abled, without three letters "dis". My mom is the reason I move forward in my life today.

Just beginning to express my feelings of love to my relatives. Grandpa and gramma would be proud of all my successes. I planted flowers on Castle Island with grandpa on September 6, 1968. I remember it like it was yesterday. I miss them both very much! Hope they see me typing from heaven!

I love all my cousins because they accept me for who I am and not my autism. But I love my mom the most. I like cousin Rose because she tried to understand me. I miss Thanksgiving and Christmas parties. I am thinking about grandpa and gramma.

Writing to Senator Kennedy, Rob said, I will ask him to see his sister Rosemary and bring her back to Hyannis to live in her home. Time to heal the past mistakes. There is nothing better than the smell of the ocean and being able to walk the shoreline with a friend or sister or brother.

Gunnar knows everything. If he says it's wrong, it is. Gunnar, you are my hero! You believe in me and I want you to know your messages of hope will be discussed forever. I admired listening to him at conferences, but most of all on his back porch. I listened and could form opinions on discussions he and mom talked about. But I could not let him know. He was right. Gunnar looked at me and did not know I could form words and be smart. Typing put me on an even keel to talk to him.

Herb (Lovett) was a man who cared about our people. He cared enough to drive to Maine to help a man. That night he died in a crash. It changed my life. Herb is still part of my circle in spirit form.

Herb was the institutional population's Christ. Here we all take a stand, that no longer will suffering be allowed! No more! No more! Herb's life needs to live in our hearts and soul.

On my Support Team

Mark has helped me through so much of the bad stuff. He helped get me out of browning road (group home). Stephen and Roger deserve mention for the continuous support they give me every day.

I am happy Stephen stayed for five years, because you care about me and treat me so special as an adult. I love the music in the morning. You can play in the afternoon and evening too. I hope the next 5 years are special.

I am glad Roger is happy. We like the garden. I believe we are ahead of schedule. There are bumps in every road. I hope the team stays together forever. Yes.

On the Institutions

I was misdiagnosed and I was put away in the Fernald penitentiary. It was a sad time in my life. I felt like a criminal the first day I was in Fernald. My crime was no one really understood autism, allergies, and sadness in my heart. I was treated like a prisoner of war. Food was lousy and I had no opportunities to make choices. I have been tested by behaviorists who wanted me to behave their way. If I was good I was given food. If I was bad, I was restrained. I was beaten and locked in dark rooms; not because I was bad, but because no one took the time to understand me. Too much useless data taken. Behaviorism failed me. I almost lost my soul.

Now comes the bad stuff. I was punched in the face and stomach at night by an evil staff person. I have flashbacks about this. But the dreams are worse. Look in my records. I was timed out because I could not tell them about x. I go back to 1984. I was beaten all night. I wanted to go home.

X was the devil of our hall. He hurt many of my friends. Where were all the advocates in 1985? Shame on Michael Dukakis. So many say they want to help but walked away. A reminder of *MIC* people — Missing In Communities, held hostage year 13 (people who are there 13 years after Rob was released) Fernald humans held against their will without a voice. I am their voice.

They hurt me at Fernald but Mark (friend and staff) protects me from evil. I have nightmares still. This is something medicine cannot cure.

I need to close this part of my life. I want to forget, but can't. I'll forget Fernald only when they bulldoze it down.

Gunnar has been a Christ to the human beings in institutions throughout the world. At times, he has been like Moses, "Let my people go!"

TO THE DMR COMMISSIONER

You take a walk in the shoes of my friends at Fernald. You may trade them in for a good pair of running shoes. They will run for freedom while you chase us. We call it freedom. They call us behaviors. I was a tough case for DMR. Look at me now.

A survivor is a person who, even though he was physically and mentally beaten, refused to give up hope. Someday I would be freed. Yes, I am a survivor.

What benefit to society is having Fernald in 1998? Help my voiceless people get the hell out of Fernald.

Community and Home

A home is where you are loved, not where you are demeaned and belittled. I am doing better since DMR let me get a life. Fernald, group home, apartment, now the house. I finally have a home I share with friends of my choosing. I am very happy I have Herb's dog. Milli Rollo Cutler. I am now independent and wishes do come true — a house and now a dog. I find it amazing that many people fight for me. If this can happen to one of the so called difficult cases in Massachusetts, it should happen for others in the system. You can't buy happiness. It is a given, or is it? I wish this question to be pondered.

We want our names to belong to our home. We want vacations, to be out in the community. No more rides to the beach (without getting out of the van). I go walk on the beach.

We need a voucher program where we control where our money is spent. Group homes are obsolete. I do not blame the staff, I blame the politicians. No vision. They need a new pair of glasses.

Positive techniques are better, safer, and most of all healthier then pain. More joy less sorrow. The sad state of affairs is that I have changed, but how do I get the vendors to give everyone a life and change their philosophy about us. Message needs to be out. No Fernald, group homes, or workshops.

RECOMMENDATIONS/CONCLUSIONS

I can help by telling parents never subject your children to behaviorism. Love those children. Children need OT and SI [occupational sensory integration therapy]. As a parent for assistance in understanding autism. Ask someone who has autism to help you. After all, I can understand by being autistic.

I believe dentists are an important part in health care for a person with autism. Imagine the pain because you got cavities from all the candy recommended by a behaviorist. When you started hitting your face — their response, more candy.

I want to stress it is better to have good therapists instead of behaviorists. We should address health issues before you send us to that funnel called workshop.

I want to talk about how to improve the life of people they serve at DMR (Department of Mental Retardation). There should be a positive progression of each client that is served. Programs should have a natural predictable flow; if not, then programs should change their teaching methods. Herb Lovett was a thinker, but a solver too. Why can't more programs use Herb's approach to life? More joy, less so. Yes

Give hope to the masses of people who need help. The chapters in my life will continue to baffle the behaviorists. Good! Calling on everyone to be a friend and not a foe to our having a life. We need to make sure our lives have meaning. We hate living just to exist.

At times I type things people don't want to hear. I want you to hear me close institutions down, give my friends something you take for granted , freedom to choose where I live and the right to communicate. But the most important thing, the right to be listened to.

Why is the way people see me important. Because I have changed! Life is becoming worthwhile. I am now a vocal person with a typewriter. I enjoy going to speak at conferences. I want to do so well. I am changing the minds of nonbelievers. But I feel sometimes my words are listened to with deaf ears.

When will the revolution on total freedom from the institutions start?

SECTION V

Family Issues

21

An Unanticipated Life:
The Impact of Lifelong Caregiving

Marty Wyngaarden Krauss
Heller School, Brandeis University, Waltham, MA

Marsha Mailick Seltzer
Waisman Center, University of Wisconsin–Madison

Introduction

This chapter discusses lessons learned from a decade of studying the gratifications and challenges of caregiving among older families of adults with mental retardation. As the title of the chapter suggests, the experience of having a son or daughter with mental retardation results in family lives that have many "unanticipated" aspects. Our research has focused on the unfolding of these unanticipated aspects, on the ways in which these parents have adapted to and been changed by their circumstances, and on the lessons that can be gleaned for families in general.

In 1988, we began a longitudinal study of 461 families who have an adult son or daughter with mental retardation living at home (Seltzer & Krauss, 1989). These parents face a unique dual challenge: they have the continuing responsibility for their son or daughter who is dependent on them for care and supervision, and they have to adapt to the manifestations and consequences of their own aging. When the study began, there was growing interest in the issues of aging for persons with mental retardation (Janicki & Wisniewski, 1985), particularly with respect to where these individuals live (Hauber, Rotegard & Bruininks, 1985), what services they needed (Janicki, Otis, Puccio, Rettig, & Jacobson, 1985), and how prepared the formal service system was to meet age-related needs (Seltzer & Krauss, 1987). There was also a recognition that there was (and still is) an "informal" service system, largely invisible to public policy analysts, that shoulders a major responsibility for the welfare of the vast majority of persons with mental retardation—the family.

Oddly, very little systematic investigation had been conducted on the experiences of families over the full lifespan. It was to this knowledge gap that our study was directed.

It is a current and historical truth that most persons with mental retardation in the US — about 85% — live with their parents. Only about 15% of the US population with mental retardation lives in licensed residential settings (Fujiura & Braddock, 1992). A great deal of research has been conducted about this 15% of adults with mental retardation who live in residential programs. This research has addressed questions such as: What are their service needs? How well are their needs being met? Under what circumstances do they develop independent living skills? What is the overall quality of their lives? However, comparable questions have not been posed about adults who live with their parents. When we began our research ten years ago, there was very little knowledge about how families manage and accommodate over time to the challenges of having a son or daughter with mental retardation living in the parental home for a lifetime.

During the past decade, a great deal has been learned about this family challenge (Fullmer, Tobin, & Smith, 1997; Hayden & Goldman, 1996; Heller & Factor, 1991; McDermott, Valentine, Anderson, Gallup, & Thompson, 1997; Seltzer & Krauss, 1994). In this chapter, we summarize our findings regarding four critical questions that have been the driving force of our research for the past decade:

1. How well have these families adapted to the challenge of lifelong caregiving?
2. What factors explain parental well-being in later life?
3. What are the forces that lead to the placement of the son or daughter out of the parental home?
4. What happens to the adult with mental retardation after the parents die?

Description of the Study

The study sample consists of 461 families who live in Wisconsin and Massachusetts, all of whom met two criteria when the study began in 1988: (1) the mother was between the ages of 55 and 85, and (2) the son or daughter with mental retardation lived at home with her. Fully 90% of the families are continuing to participate in our research ten years later. Since the study began, all 461 families have experienced changes. Some have experienced dramatic changes, such as the death of the mother or father or the placement of the adult with retardation out of the home. Other families have experienced smaller changes, such as declining health in the parents or the decision to put the adult's name on a waiting list for placement.

In order to learn about these changes and their consequences, we visit each family every 18 months. At each visit, the mother participates in an in-depth interview and then is asked to complete a self-administered questionnaire of standardized measures. Information is also collected from the father and twice we have collected data from a sibling in the family. Having multiple respondents from each family provides a full-family picture of individual and family well-being, the major life events that have occurred during the past 18 months, and the changes that are expected in the near-term future. In total, each family will participate in eight rounds of data collection between 1988, when the study began, and the year 2000, when the study will be completed. A family continues in our study even when the parents are no longer living, as a sibling or another relative takes over as the primary research respondent. This is because the most riveting question that motivates parents to participate in our study is "what will happen to my son or daughter after I die?"

The average age of the mothers in our sample was 66 years in 1988 when the study began, and they ranged in age from 55 to 85. About two-thirds were married, and virtually all of the others were widows. About one-quarter still worked in a paid position outside of the home, even though most were of retirement age. Their adult sons and daughters with retardation averaged 33 years of age. There was an enormous spread in their ages, ranging from the youngest who was 15 years of age in 1988, to the oldest who was age 66 at that time. Most — about 80% — had mild or moderate mental retardation. About one-third had Down syndrome. Fully 90% of these adults had a job or a vocational day placement, giving their parents a regular break from the demands of caregiving.

Findings: What Have We Learned?

HOW WELL HAVE THESE FAMILIES ADAPTED TO THE CHALLENGES OF LIFELONG CAREGIVING?

When the study began, we hypothesized that, after an average of nearly 35 years of active parenting for a son or daughter with a disability, the mothers in these families would have compromised well-being. Because of the centrality of mothers in the caregiving arrangements, they were the primary focus of our study. We expected that their long years of caregiving would take a toll on them and that they would feel more burdened and depressed than other women their age. It also was expected that the challenge of having a child with a disability and the extra time that caregiving takes every day of their lives would limit the social activities and contacts of these mothers, as compared with their age peers who did not have such responsibilities.

However, the data did not support these hypotheses. Despite the long period of active parenting, mothers have a very favorable level of personal and social well-being (Krauss & Seltzer, 1993). We compared our data with data on several other groups of women and found that the mothers in our study have no greater parenting stress than mothers of younger children with retardation. Also, they report no greater level of subjective burden than caregivers of elderly relatives. They have comparable levels of life satisfaction and no greater risk of depression than other women their age who have not had lifelong caregiving responsibilities. And they have social support networks that are comparable in size to the networks that other older women enjoy.

These are pretty remarkable findings in light of the many demands that these mothers have faced during their decades of caregiving, the challenge of having a child with a disability, and the fundamental difference in their life course as compared with the lives of women whose children did not have disabilities. These findings challenge the conventional stereotype of — and our initial hypothesis about — the impact of lifelong caregiving.

Stepping back in time, however, it is recognized that when a child with mental retardation is first diagnosed, parents almost universally react to the news with deep grief and disappointment. How is this tragedy transformed into a challenge that can be coped with? Here is an account of how one mother in our study described her experiences after her daughter was born (Hegeman, 1984). She wrote this in 1953, when her daughter was 6 years old.

> Virginia was born when I was 36 years of age, our first and only child. I had an easy and pleasant delivery, being awake during it all and conversing with the doctor. My first questions after the delivery were "Is she all right? Does she have all her fingers and toes?" The doctor said that she had. I was taken back to my room. But about 20 minutes later the doctor came in with tears streaming down his cheeks. He said, "Mrs. Wing, I was wrong. I hadn't noticed it immediately after your baby was born, but there is *something terribly wrong* with the baby."
>
> He couldn't tell me at first. I took hold of his hands and begged him to tell me. He finally told me that my baby was the type known as 'Mongoloid.' I had never heard the term before, and it struck absolute terror into my whole body.
>
> I asked the doctor many questions: If these children ever walked, or talked, or if they were complete idiots. Would they look funny? Would they have to be cared for as babies all their lives? And many more. The doctor did not have answers.
>
> I was completely terrified over the situation. I never closed my eyes in sleep for about three months, except for about one hour every night, and then I would awaken and immediately think, "Virginia is an idiot, an idiot, an idiot.." I would be so terrified until morning came that I don't know how my mind remained firm.

Virginia's mother went on to describe the depths of her despair and depression. Her account was published in a textbook, which she was asked to update almost 35 years later in 1987, one year before she joined our study. At the time of this update, Virginia was about 40 years of age. Her mother's concluding words in the update were:

> Suffice it to say that our family has prospered. Virginia is now the joy of our family, and without her our lives would seem empty and have less meaning.

What transforms an event that was initially felt to be such a great tragedy into a source of joy and pride for these families? What are the processes and mechanisms that account for the overall positive outcomes that we have observed in these mothers, even though they have lived with extraordinary challenges for decades? These are the central questions that have driven and continue to drive our study. We are lucky to have access to two perspectives on how the transformation from "tragedy" to "pride and joy" takes place, one based on the parents' subjective and retrospective accounts, and the other based on prospective, empirical analyses that have been guided by general social and psychological theories. We focus first on parents' retrospective accounts of why and how they have managed so well, and then to turn to our prospective, theoretically-driven analyses of the factors that have led to these favorable outcomes.

WHAT FACTORS EXPLAIN FAMILY WELL-BEING IN LATER LIFE?

Based on the retrospective accounts provided by the mothers, three processes that *they believe* helped them to adapt to the challenges of lifelong caregiving have been identified. First, many of these mothers reported that they *altered their values* and redefined what they hold important in life. One mother commented,

> I am well aware of the price I paid to be a full-time mother to our son. It cost me the opportunity for a career and what might have been a good education. But he was worth it, and I'd make the same choices again.

Second, many mothers feel that having a child with a disability gave them *a mission to work for*. When these children were born, in the early to mid-1950s, it was more common than it is today for women to stay at home to raise a family. Many had tremendous untapped potential for leadership and creativity. Having a child with a disability gave some of these women an avenue to channel their energies and resources. This is the generation of parents who organized The Arc movement, who brought class action lawsuits that resulted in the deinstitutionalization movement, and who lobbied for legislation to guarantee their children an education like all other children. For some of the women in our study, this special mission transformed their lives.

For example, one mother in our study recalled that over 30 years ago, she was a college student, hoping to become a teacher. Then her son with Down syndrome was born. She dropped out of college to take care of John. After a difficult period of adjustment, not very different from that of Virginia=s mother, John's mother joined the League of Women Voters. She became active in local politics, and after several years she decided to run for public office. She was elected mayor of her town, a position that she held for 17 years. She attributes her success in politics to John, her son with Down syndrome. She said that her initial aspirations for a career as a teacher were far surpassed by her achievements in politics. She feels that having a son with Down syndrome helped her to break out of the mold and to stretch herself to her fullest potential. Other mothers, who have not had such a visible public profile, have a similar sense of how their special parenting challenge has helped them to achieve more than they would have otherwise. One mother noted,

> It gave direction to my life and gave me something to work for. It also became a positive force for others. In helping my own daughter find a niche in the world, I also inadvertently helped other families to do the same for their children.

The third process that these mothers felt helped them in their life journey was the *reciprocity of the relationship* with their son or daughter. Help flows in many directions in these families. Especially when the parents are in old age and are increasingly frail, having a healthy son or daughter living at home can be a wonderful resource. One mother explained that in the early years after her daughter's birth, were it not for her husband, she would never have been able to care for her daughter with retardation at home. But now her husband has Alzheimer's disease, and were it not for her daughter's help, she would have to place her husband in a nursing home. Together, she and her daughter care for her husband, just as she and her husband had cared for their daughter earlier in life. So these families travel through life together, exchanging assistance and support. It is simplistic to think of the parents only as caregivers, as we have seen many examples of how they *receive help from* — as well as *give help to* — their son or daughter with the disability. One mother which sums up the experience of many in our study:

> Having a retarded child is a terrible tragedy, but I wouldn't trade him for any normal child. If one can get beyond the grief and sorrow about what he has lost — and that takes some doing — then experiencing life through his eyes and sharing a life with him so filled with joy and innocence has been an extraordinary path to take. I wouldn't have missed it for the world.

We also looked to the general behavioral and social science literature for theories to help guide our examination of the processes by which these families manage the stresses of their lives. One applicable paradigm is the stress and coping model, articulated by Pearlin and colleagues (Pearlin, Mullan, Semple, & Skaff, 1990; Pearlin & Schooler, 1978). They have argued that under conditions of high stress, individuals can maintain their psychological well-being by using effective coping strategies, which can reduce distress by resolving the problem.

More specifically, the stress and coping model posits that when people are faced with stressful situations, they are able to avoid psychological distress if they use problem-focused coping strategies and if they refrain from using emotion-focused coping. Problem-focused coping involves cognitive and behavioral strategies aimed at altering or managing the stressful situation. For example, problem-focused coping includes coping by planning ahead, actively trying to solve the problem, setting other challenges aside to deal with the problem, and reinterpreting the problem in a positive light (Folkman & Lazarus, 1980). Past research on the general population has revealed that by working to solve the problem, people can reduce their feelings of distress that arise in response to stressful situations (Pratt et al., 1985). Emotion-focused coping, on the other hand, involves cognitive and behavioral efforts to reduce or manage emotional distress, but which are not focused directly on solving or altering the problem. For example, emotion-focused coping includes coping by strategies as diverse as venting and expressing the emotions that accompany a problematic situation and disengaging from or denying the problem. Despite these attempts to manage emotional distress, past research has revealed that using emotion-focused coping strategies generally does not result in improved well-being (Haley et al, 1987; Kramer, 1993). Rather, over time, using emotion-focused coping appears to *fuel* psychological distress.

We tested the applicability of Pearlin's stress and coping model to aging mothers of adults with mental retardation by investigating whether these mothers, when faced with high levels of caregiving challenges, could maintain their psychological well-being by using problem-focused coping strategies and by avoiding the use of emotion-focused coping. The two stressful situations we investigated were high levels of caregiving demands and severe behavior problems in the son or daughter.

Specifically, we found that similar to the patterns evident in the general population, when the aging mothers in our sample had a son or daughter with high levels of caregiving demands or severe behavior problems, they could avoid depressive symptoms if they relied on problem-focused coping strategies (Seltzer, Greenberg, & Krauss, 1995). We also found that mothers who relied on emotion-focused coping showed an elevated level of depressive symptoms regardless of their level of stress.

During the course of our decade-long study, we have found through longitudinal analyses that these effects gradually accumulate over time. So, using effective coping strategies in the face of stress is one way that aging mothers with lifelong caregiving responsibilities have successfully regulated their psychological well-being over the many decades of caregiving.

In addition to adaptive coping, the effectiveness of other normative processes that may have contributed to the positive well-being profiles of the mothers in their adaptation to their non-normative life circumstance has been investigated. One of these processes concerns the extent to which mothers are engaged in multiple roles, and whether involvement in multiple roles leads to positive outcomes (Sieber, 1974; Thoits, 1986) or instead to role overload (Marks, 1977; Repetti, Matthews & Waldron, 1989). It is important to note that researchers and service providers in the field of developmental disabilities may focus in on only one aspect of these women's lives, namely their role as a mother of an adult with mental retardation. The fact that they occupy other roles that may be equally as important to them and that may be even more influential in shaping their psychological well-being is too often ignored. Other roles commonly held by women in later life include formal roles such as employee, caregiver for another relative or a friend, and volunteer, and also the informal and familial roles of spouse, parent, grandparent, friend, relative, and neighbor.

The role overload hypothesis predicts that mothers who have ongoing caregiving responsibilities for an adult with mental retardation would find the demands of many other roles to be overwhelming, leading to declining psychological well-being (Marks, 1997; Repetti, Matthews, & Waldron, 1989). The alternative hypothesis posits that holding multiple roles may have a positive effect, serving as a source of social integration, social support, and self-esteem, which consequently may lead to better psychological well-being (Sieber, 1974; Thoits, 1983). The literature on the general population supports the benefits of holding multiple roles (Adelmann, 1994; Pietromonaco, Manis & Frohardt-Lane, 1986).

We examined these two competing hypotheses about the effects of holding multiple roles (Hong & Seltzer, 1995). Similar to normative processes in the general population, aging mothers of adults with retardation who hold multiple roles have better psychological well-being than those with a more constricted range of social roles. In addition, in longitudinal analyses, we found that increasing the number of roles held, even during the later decades of the life course, led to increases in psychological well-being (Hong, 1996). In other words, mothers who got a new job, or who became newly involved with their neighborhood association, for example, evidenced an increase in psychological well-being as compared with their prior state. These longitudinal analyses controlled for prior levels of well-being, which suggested that the multiple role effect was independent of the benefit of previous levels of mental health.

In addition to these findings regarding coping and multiple role effects, we investigated how social support may influence the psychological well-being of the mothers in our sample. Based on longitudinal analyses, we found that social support has a measurable effect on change in maternal well-being (Greenberg, Seltzer,

Krauss, & Kim, 1997). Furthermore, there is evidence regarding different effects of social support at different stages of life. We found that for mothers in their *60s,* having a social support network that expanded or grew during a five-year period led to improved psychological well-being. For women in their *70s and 80s,* the salient aspect of social support was not the number of friends and close relatives, as it was for their counterparts in their 60s, but rather receiving increasing amounts of emotional support (Hong & Seltzer, 1998). For these two age cohorts, having a larger social network and more emotional support, respectively, were associated with increasingly favorable well-being profiles.

Together, these analyses suggest that aging mothers of adults with retardation — a group of women who have provided hands-on care to their son or daughter for decades, who have not had the opportunity to experience the empty nest stage of life with its concomitant freedom to retire on their own terms, and who have trepidation about the future quality of life of their son or daughter after they are no longer the primary caregiver — actually have a great deal of *control* over their level of psychological well-being. They are less depressed and have more positive mental health when they do three things:

1. Use problem-focused coping strategies when faced with high levels of caregiving stress, and avoid emotion-focused coping,
2. Remain vitally engaged in the multiple roles of life, rather than reducing their role involvement in order to care for their son or daughter with mental retardation, and
3. Maintain their social relationships and continue to develop new relationships with people who can be a source of emotional support to them even in their 60s, 70s, and 80s.

Under these circumstances, women with ongoing caregiving responsibilities are not highly distressed and instead have surprisingly positive well-being profiles. It is important to keep in mind the generalizability of these processes, particularly in light of the atypicality of their life situations.

Do the qualitative and the quantitative components of our study imply similar or different processes about adaptation? Although the mothers do not conceptualize their well-being in social and behavioral science terms, the validity of these processes in the subjective experiences of the mothers is confirmed in our analyses. Regarding problem-focused coping, recall the mother who commented that having a child with retardation

> gave direction to my life and gave me something to work for... In helping my own daughter find a niche in the world, I also inadvertently helped other families to do the same for their children.

By coping adaptively, this mother was able to feel good about making a difference in her daughter's life as well as contributing to the well-being of other families.

Regarding multiple roles, recall the mother who became the mayor of her city and who became a political force at the same time that she provided daily care to her son with Down syndrome. By maintaining multiple roles, this mother stretched her capacities to the fullest, developed a healthy sense of self-esteem, and avoided focusing only on the difficulties faced by her son with mental retardation.

Regarding social support, recall that these families are from the generation which founded the Arc, and which developed parent support groups (Dybwad, 1990). The Arc gave them a locus of support which helped them to maintain their psychological well-being, gave them a feeling of solidarity with others in a similar life circumstance, and thus avoided feelings of isolation.

These are the stories and the mechanisms which explain the overall pattern of success that we have found, and that have helped us to understand why parenting a son or daughter with retardation for a lifetime generally does not result in the tragic outcomes that parents initially imagine or were often told to expect. Having followed these families for a decade, the patterns just described appear to be characteristic of the lives of these parents during their later years of active parenting. However, we also have found that the patterns persist only as long as the mothers, in particular, are in reasonably good health and are able to maintain their coping abilities, their multiple roles, and their social contacts.

WHAT ARE THE FACTORS THAT LEAD TO THE PLACEMENT OF THE SON OR DAUGHTER OUT OF THE PARENTAL HOME?

We also have investigated the factors that lead to the end of the time when the parents and the adult with retardation live together in the same home — the end of lifelong caregiving. This is an *inevitable ending* in all families, unless the son or daughter with retardation dies before the parents. Some parents view placement into a community residential setting in a positive light, as an opportunity for their son or daughter to become more independent and live a more adult life.

One mother who held this positive view explained,

> We are very happy with him at home, but we do feel we need to prepare for the future. That's why we put his name on the waiting list.

This is an example of one type of problem-focused coping, namely planning ahead.

However, for most parents, this is a transition about which there is deep-seated ambivalence and fear, and which many wish they could avoid. As we have reported elsewhere (Essex, Seltzer & Krauss, 1997; Freedman, Krauss & Seltzer, 1997), fewer than half of the families in our study — about 45% — have made long range plans, either putting the adult=s name on a waiting list for residential placement or planning that siblings or other relatives will take the adult with retardation into their own home. However, the majority of *even* those who had made concrete plans for placement hope that their adult child will remain at home for the foreseeable future. This translates into less than a quarter of the families in our study who have *both* made a plan for their adult son or daughter's residential placement *and* hope that the placement will occur soon.

What happens to the plans made by families? Are these plans implemented? Do they influence the long-term future of the son or daughter for whom the plans are made? Our analyses reveal that planning does not always — or even, often — work out exactly the way the parents would like it to. That is because the service system in most states is not equipped to respond to the many adults with mental retardation who need to or would prefer to live away from the parental home. At the present time, there are approximately 87,000 adults with mental retardation on formal waiting lists for a residential placement in the US, most of whom are currently living with their parents (Lakin, 1998; Prouty & Lakin, 1997). Therefore, parents who plan ahead by adding their child=s name to a waiting list generally have to wait for a very long time.

Our data show that there are three different routes to placement (Essex, Seltzer & Krauss, 1997). Some parents want their son or daughter to make this lifestyle change while they, the parents, are still well enough *to help ease the transition* with their support. Their goal is to complete the transition before they, the parents, encounter the age-related problems they all fear. These parents are prepared to wait for several years until the funding can be arranged for their son or daughter to move to a residential placement of their choice.

A second factor that sets placement into motion is *health problems in the son or daughter*. Older adults with retardation often have health problems of their own, and they may need more physical care than their elderly parents can provide. In particular, adults with Down syndrome are at risk for early-onset aging, which may involve dementia and other health difficulties. These health problems sometimes get to the point where nursing care is needed.

In yet other families, *an emergency propels the placement.* In such cases, a new living arrangement for the son or daughter with the disability can be found in a matter of hours. In fact, we found that a health emergency in the mother is the single greatest predictor of the residential placement of her son or daughter. Here is an extreme example of a placement propelled by an emergency.

In this family, the mother was a widow, and her daughter with severe retardation lived with her. There was a grown brother who lived near the mother, and a sister who lived in a nearby city. The brother was a prominent banker. The mother began to develop the symptoms of Alzheimer's disease. Her ability to run her own household and take care of her daughter with mental retardation began to be impaired. During one of the routine visits by the banker to his mother, he realized that the situation had reached a crisis and he concluded that his mother and his sister were no longer safe living at home together. The banker quickly began to make arrangements for his mother to enter a nursing home. Once this plan was implemented, he put his sister into the car along with her belongings which were stuffed into a large plastic garbage bag. The banker then drove his sister to a public agency that served persons with mental retardation. He demanded that the agency find a new home for his sister immediately. And then he drove away, leaving his sister behind. The banker's actions were widely criticized in the newspapers, given his high public profile and his ample financial means. But, a residential placement was found for the sister within a few hours.

Regardless of the route to placement, about 25% of the adults in our study now are living away from their parents' home, for many for the first time in their lives (Seltzer, Greenberg, Krauss, & Hong, 1997). Where do these adults live? The vast majority (about 70%) of the adults who have moved away from their parents' home have moved to supervised community living, either a group home, fully staffed apartment, or foster home. About 15% live either independently or semi-independently in the community. However, it was disturbing to see that nearly 10% moved to an institutional setting or to a nursing home. Finally, only 5% are living with family, primarily their siblings.

Thus, only a minority of families anticipate the transition of the adult out of the parental home as a positive developmental stage in life. Rather, most fear this transition, and fewer than half make concrete plans for it. Even when plans are made, long waiting lists in almost every state limit access to residential placements. However, we have found that, in an emergency, placements can be made in a matter of hours. Nevertheless, when placement does occur, either due to an emergency or because of effective advance planning, most adults live in community-based settings.

WHAT HAPPENS TO THE ADULT WITH RETARDATION AFTER THE PARENTS DIE?

Lastly, we addressed a question that is, for many parents, the most difficult question they ponder, namely what will happen to their son or daughter when they are no longer alive and able to provide care. Questions that haunt them include, "Where will my daughter live?" "Who will take care of her?" "How can her quality of life be maintained?" "Will my other children be able to help their sister without sacrificing their own lives?" These persistent and nagging questions affect all family members — parents and siblings alike — and also are a concern to many adults with retardation.

It is important to note that, as recently as a generation ago, these questions were not frequently on parents' minds because it was much more common than it is today for children with mental retardation to die before their parents. So the present generation of older parents have few role models to guide them as they think ahead about the future.

In our sample of 461 families, a death of one parent has occurred in 234 families. In 38 of these families, both parents are now deceased, whereas in the others, one parent remains alive. This is a large enough group to gauge the answer to the parents' question, "What will happen to my child after I die?"

We have found that after the death of *one parent*, the surviving parent generally assumes the caregiving responsibilities of the other parent (Gordon, Seltzer & Krauss, 1997). The transmission of caregiving responsibility, not surprisingly, is more difficult when the surviving parent is the father. This is because prior to the death of the mother, most fathers in our sample generally provided very little hands-on daily care to their adult child. But after the death of the mother, we have found that nearly all surviving fathers in our sample have taken on this role.

Placement in a residential setting is *not* a frequent response to the death of one parent, as long as the other parent remains alive. It is almost as if the surviving parent cannot bear the prospect of losing a second close family member in such a short period of time. This is one instance where mutual support and reciprocal caregiving is often seen — where the adult with retardation is a source of emotional and practical support to the widowed mother or father, while at the same time he or she receives support from this parent.

Ultimately, however, these adults must face the loss of both of their parents. This is a very different transition than the loss of just one parent. When both parents die, a change in the adult's living arrangement is needed. In our study, about three-fourths of the adults who have lost both parents moved to a residential placement. The other quarter moved in with relatives, usually a sibling (Krauss, Seltzer, Gordon, & Friedman, 1996). When the death of the second parent is sudden, it is generally the case that a temporary arrangement has to be worked out until a satisfactory longer-term residential plan can be put into place.

We have seen that the death of both parents sets into motion an enormous range of changes in the life circumstances of adults with mental retardation. Of course, there is a change in where these adults live. In addition, in most cases this involves a change in job or day activity. Their primary source of emotional support is gone. Their social life changes. This transition is truly a crisis in the life of an adult with mental retardation.

Summary and Conclusions

After 10 years of studying aging in families with an adult with mental retardation, we are more convinced than ever that society has much to learn from these families and from similar families everywhere. Most of all, *these families should be respected*. They should be honored for their commitment to provide a loving home for their son or daughter well into adulthood, for changing their personal priorities, and for restructuring their family lifestyles. And they should be *understood with compassion* when they worry about the future. In the words of one mother,

> Our major problem remains the same as it has been since his birth — who will care for him when we cannot? Caring for him ourselves, adjusting our lifestyles, is manageable — can even be very rewarding. It is the worry about his uncertain future that is *the* problem for us.

At times, the bonds between these parents and their adult child may seem extraordinarily close. Perhaps these bonds are what it takes to sustain family-based care over many decades. Here are the words of one father:

> Although he is retarded and physically handicapped ... there would be a serious void in our lives if he were no longer with us. He has done as much to enrich our lives as we have done to enrich his. We don't regret for one minute the fact that my wife gave birth to an 'abnormal' human being. *He is us!*

Lastly, we should learn from these families that effective coping may ultimately rest on the ability to reflect on core values and redefine what is important in life. In the words of one mother:

> This child taught me an appreciation for the little things in life that we all take for granted. My other children learned about love and caring for others from Cindy. I don't ask 'Why me?" I ask, 'Why *not* me?'

References

Adelmann, P.K. (1994). Multiple roles and psychological well-being in a national sample of older adults. *Journal of Gerontology: Social Science, 49,* 277-285.

Dybwad, R.F. (1990). *Perspectives on a parent movement.* Cambridge, MA: Brookline Books.

Essex, E.L., Seltzer, M.M., & Krauss, M.W. (1997). Residential transitions of adults with mental retardation: Predictors of waiting list use and placement. *American Journal on Mental Retardation, 101,* 613-629.

Folkman, S., & Lazarus, R.S. (1980). An analysis of coping in a middle-aged community sample. *Journal of Health and Social Behavior, 21,* 219-239.

Freedman, R.I., Krauss, M.W., & Seltzer, M.M. (1997). Aging parents' residential plans for adult children with mental retardation. *Mental Retardation, 35,* 114-123.

Fujiura, G.T., & Braddock, D. (1992). Fiscal and demographic trends in mental retardation services: The emergence of the family. In L. Rowitz (Ed.), *Mental retardation in the year 2000.* New York: Springer-Verlag.

Fullmer, E.M., Tobin, S.S., & Smith, G.C. (1997). The effects of offspring gender on older mothers caring for their sons and daughters with mental retardation. *The Gerontologist, 37,* 795-803.

Gordon, R.M., Seltzer, M.M., & Krauss, M.W. (1997). The aftermath of parental death: Changes in the context and quality of life. In R. L. Schalock (Ed.) *Quality of life, Volume II - Application to persons with disabilities* (pp. 25-42). Washington, D.C.: American Association on Mental Retardation.

Greenberg, J.S., Seltzer, M.M., Krauss, M.W., & Kim, H. (1997). The differential effects of social support on the psychological well-being of aging mothers of adults with mental illness or mental retardation. *Family Relations, 46*, 383-394.

Haley, W.E., Levine, E.G., Brown, S.C., & Bartolucci, A.A. (1987). Stress, appraisal, coping, and social support as predictors of adaptational outcomes among dementia caregivers. *Psychology and Aging, 2*, 323-330.

Hauber, F.A., Rotegard, L.L., & Bruininks, R.H. (1985). Characteristics of residential services for older/elderly mentally retarded persons. In M. P. Janicki & H. M. Wisniewski (Eds.) *Aging and developmental disabilities: Issues and Approaches* (pp. 327-350). Baltimore, MD: Brookes.

Hayden, M. F., & Goldman, J. (1996). Families of adults with mental retardation: Stress levels and need for services. *Social Work, 41*, 657-667.

Hegeman, M.T. (1984). *Developmental disability: A family challenge.* New York: Paulist Press.

Heller, T. & Factor, A. (1991). Permanency planning for adults with mental retardation living with family caregivers. *American Journal on Mental Retardation, 96*, 163-176.

Hong, J. (1996). *Are they the blessedly stressed, too? A study of multiple roles and psychological well-being among older and caregiving women.* Ph.D. dissertation, Department of Sociology, University of Wisconsin-Madison, Madison, WI.

Hong, J., & Seltzer, M.M. (1998). *Stability and change in the social support of older women: A longitudinal study of psychological well-being.* (Manuscript submitted for publication.)

Hong, J., & Seltzer, M.M. (1995). The psychological consequences of multiple roles: The nonnormative case. *Journal of Health and Social Behavior, 36*, 386-398.

Janicki, M.P., Otis, J.P., Puccio, P.S., Rettig, J.H., & Jacobson, J.W. (1985). Service needs among older developmentally disabled persons. In M. P. Janicki & H. M. Wisniewski (Eds.) *Aging and developmental disabilities: Issues and approache* (pp. 289-304). Baltimore, MD: Brookes.

Janicki, M.P., & Wisniewski, H.M. (Eds.) (1985). *Aging and developmental disabilities: Issues and approaches.* Baltimore, MD: Brookes.

Krauss, M.W., & Seltzer, M.M. (1993). Coping strategies among older mothers of adults with retardation: A life span developmental perspective. In A.P. Turnbull, J.M. Patterson, S.K. Behr, D.L. Murphy, J.G. Marquis, & M.J. Blue-Banning (Eds.), *Cognitive coping, families, and disability* (pp. 173-182). Baltimore, MD: Brookes.

Krauss, M.W., Seltzer, M.M., Gordon, R., & Friedman, D.H. (1996). Binding ties: The roles of adult siblings of persons with mental retardation. *Mental Retardation, 34*, 83-93.

Lakin, K.C. (1998). On the outside looking in: Attending to waiting lists in systems of services for people with developmental disabilities. *Mental Retardation, 36*, 157-162.

Marks, S.R. (1977). Multiple roles and role strain: Some notes on human energy, time, and commitment. *American Sociological Review, 42*, 247-260.

McDermott, S., Valentine, D., Anderson, D., Gallup, D., & Thompson, S. (1997). Parents of adults with mental retardation living in-home and out-of-home: Caregiving burdens and gratifications. *American Journal of Orthopsychiatry, 67*, 323-329.

Pearlin, L.I., Mullan, J.T., Semple, S.J., & Skaff, M.M. (1990). Caregiving and the stress process: An overview of concepts and their measures. *The Gerontologist, 30*, 583-594.

Pearlin, L., & Schooler, C. (1978). The structure of coping. *Journal of Health and Social Behavior, 19*, 2-21.

Pietromonaco, P.R., Manis, J., & Frohardt-Lane, K. (1986). Psychological consequences of multiple social roles. *Psychology of Women Quarterly, 10*, 373-382.

Pratt, C., Schmall,V., Wright, S., & Cleveland, M. (1985). Burden and coping strategies of caregivers to Alzheimer=s patients. *Family Relations, 34*, 27-33.

Prouty, R.W., & Lakin, K.C. (Eds.). (1997). *Residential services for persons with developmental disabilities. Status and trends through 1996.* Minneapolis: University of Minnesota, Research & Training Center on Community Living/Institute on Community Integration.

Repetti, R.L., Matthews, K.A., & Waldron, I. (1989). Effects of paid employment on women=s mental and physical health. *American Psychologist, 44*, 1394-1401.

Seltzer, M.M. & Krauss, M.W. (1987). *Aging and mental retardation: Extending the continuum.* Washington, DC: American Association on Mental Retardation, Monograph Series, Monograph No. 9.

Seltzer, M.M., & Krauss, M.W. (1989). Aging parents with mentally retarded children: Family risk factors and sources of support. *American Journal on Mental Retardation, 94,* 303-312.

Seltzer, M.M., & Krauss, M.W. (1994). Aging parents with co-resident adult children: The impact of lifelong caregiving. In M.M. Seltzer, M.W. Krauss, & M.P. Janicki (Eds.), *Life course perspectives on adulthood and old age* (pp. 3-18). Washington, D.C.: The American Association on Mental Retardation Monograph Series.

Seltzer, M.M., Greenberg, J.S., & Krauss, M.W. (1995). A comparison of coping strategies of aging mothers of adults with mental illness or mental retardation. *Psychology and Aging, 10,* 64-75.

Seltzer, M.M., Greenberg, J.S., Krauss, M.W., & Hong, J. (1997). Predictors and outcomes of the end of co-resident caregiving in aging families of adults with mental retardation or mental illness. *Family Relations, 46,* 13-22.

Sieber, S.D. (1974). Toward a theory of role accumulation. *American Sociological Review, 39,* 567-578.

Thoits, P.A. (1986). Multiple identities: Examining gender and marital status differences in distress. *American Sociological Review, 51,* 259-272.

22

Gender, Disability, and Community Life
Toward a Feminist Analysis

Rannveig Traustadóttir
University of Iceland, Reykjavik, Iceland

Gender and gender asymmetry are fundamental aspects of social life. In feminist writings gender is most commonly regarded as a system of culturally constructed relations of power (Lorber & Farrell, 1991; Richardson & Taylor,1993; Tong, 1998). The constant construction and reconstruction of gender relations is an integral part of every society's structure of domination and subordination. Gender relations influence the division of labor in the family and the labor market, and gender, as a social status, shapes the individual's opportunities for education, employment, family, sexuality, authority, and the possibility to make an impact on the production of culture. Societies vary in the extent to which women and men are unequal, but where there is inequality woman are invariably devalued and allocated work that is also devalued, whether it is paid or unpaid. Gender is intertwined with other socially constructed categories of differential evaluation such as race and disability. Despite this, few attempts have been made to examine the interconnection between gender and disability and how gender has influenced the current reforms in the field of developmental disabilities.

In this chapter I examine how gender relations influence issues of disability by providing a feminist analysis of the current reform toward full inclusion of people with disabilities into everyday community life. Feminist approaches are varied and diverse (see for example Tong, 1998) but much of today's feminist analysis is characterized by the emphasis on the importance of acknowledging the pervasive influence of gender and attempts to uncover the links between gender and other asymmetric systems (Richardson & Taylor, 1993). A feminist critique of current policies and practices in the developmental disability field provides an alternative view of the reform and a new framework to understand the everyday realities of the people who have been most influenced by it: women and men with disabilities, their families, and the human service workers who carry out the daily work of inclusion and acceptance of people with disabilities.

Examining issues of gender as well as other social dimensions such as culture, class, race, ethnicity, and sexuality, enables us to move beyond the medical approach to disability and the white middle class male bias and compartmentalization that has characterized much of the research and writing in the field. This new approach to studying disability attempts to provide a more accurate understanding of the lived experiences of all those affected by disability and more sophisticated methods to unravel the complex social, political, and cultural forces that influence our lives.

The deinstitutionalization movement started in the 1970s in most western industrialized countries (Scheerenberger, 1983; 1987). In the early days, the reform efforts focused on moving people with developmental disabilities out of large total institutions. Later, the emphasis has been on the social participation of people with disabilities in everyday community life (Taylor, Bogdan, & Knoll, 1987). Today, a quarter of a century later, this humanistic reform is still on going. Countries around the world are at different stages in their efforts to include people with disabilities in all aspects of community life. However, implementing community inclusion has proven to be much slower and, in particular, more complicated than expected. Most countries are still struggling with closing down segregated services and developing new community-based programs (Bradley, Ashbaugh, & Blaney, 1994; Hayden & Abery, 1994; Sandvin, 1993; Sandvin, Söder, Lichtwarck, & Magnussen, 1998; Taylor, Biklen, & Knoll, 1987; Tøssebro, Gustavsson, & Dyredal, 1996). Thus, the reform is still in progress and there is reason to believe that the goal of full inclusion of all people with disabilities in all aspects of community life is far in the future.

Researchers, policy makers, professionals, and service providers are struggling to understand why the reform is going so slowly and why it has proven so difficult to fulfil the promise of full inclusion. Some have pointed out that the obstacles may partly derive from the fact that research, as well as policies and practices, in the field of developmental disability have traditionally been narrowly focused on issues of disability and have, for the most part, ignored other social dimensions (Fine & Asch, 1988; Traustadóttir, 1992; Traustadóttir, Lutfiyya, & Shoultz, 1994). The field also seems to have an over-simplified understanding of community life and the social, political, and cultural dynamics that influence the implementation of community inclusion. We need a more sophisticated understanding of the forces that influence the participation of people with disabilities in everyday community life. We need to understand the interconnections between disability and other categories of inequality, such as gender, so that the relationship amongst categories of inequality can inform our policies and practices in the field of disability.

The feminist analysis provided in this chapter highlights how important it is that we broaden our view beyond issues of disability when discussing community inclusion. Traditionally, people in the field have focused on the impairment when anticipating what would be the greatest obstacles to community participation and have assumed that people with the most severe disabilities would have the greatest difficulties in gaining acceptance as community members. This narrow focus on the disability, as the crucial issue in community integration, has prevented us from identifying other social factors, such as gender, which may be equally important.

This analysis of community inclusion is part of a growing movement in the field of developmental disabilities to broaden the horizons to include an examination of how disability intersects with social issues such as class, race, culture, gender, sexuality, and ethnicity (Bérubé, 1996; Brown & Smith, 1992; Fadiman, 1997; Fine & Asch, 1988; Harry, 1992; Kalyanpur & Rao, 1991; Lynch & Hansen, 1992; O'Connor, 1992; 1993; Wilson, O'Reilly & Russ, 1991).

A comprehensive feminist analysis of the field of developmental disability and the current reforms is beyond the scope of this chapter. This analysis is limited to examining how gender may be influencing three aspects of community inclusion of people with disabilities. First, I examine gender and community participation of women and men with disabilities, in particular, how disability policies and practices affect the lives of women and men in different ways. Secondly, I provide an analysis of families of children with disabilities and the gendered division of caring in these families. Third, I examine the human services system and the gendered organization of caring work in disability services. The theme uniting these three areas is the emphasis on understanding how issues of gender influence the current reforms and the everyday lives of people with disabilities, their families, friends, and the people who work in the field.

GENDER AND COMMUNITY PARTICIPATION OF WOMEN AND MEN WITH DISABILITIES

Gender is built into the social order in many crucial ways. The major social institutions of control—law, medicine, religion, politics—treat women and men differently, generally discriminating against women and men of disadvantaged groups. Thus, while both women and men with disabilities are subject to discrimination because of their disabilities, women with disabilities are at a further disadvantage because of the combined discrimination based on gender and on disability (Asch & Fine, 1988; Morris, 1996; Traustadóttir, 1997a).

Most disability research has assumed the irrelevance of gender when addressing the lives and experiences of people with disabilities and their possibilities to participate in everyday community life. Instead, the obstacles people with disabilities may meet have been explained by their impairments. When considering the possibility of community participation of people with disabilities the discourse of "level of disability" has been dominant and it has been commonly assumed that people with the most severe disabilitie,s will have the greatest difficulties in gaining acceptance as community members. This emphasis on the disability as the most crucial issue in community participation has prevented us from identifying other social dimensions, such as culture, class, race, ethnicity, sexual orientation, and gender, as equally important (Traustadóttir, Lutfiyya, & Shoultz, 1994). "Having a disability presumably eclipses these dimensions of social experience. Even sensitive studies of disability ... have focused on disability as a unitary concept and have taken it to be not merely the 'master' status, but apparently the exclusive status for disabled people" (Asch & Fine, 1988: 3).

Feminist research has demonstrated how gender influences non-disabled people's participation in different spheres of society. In particular, feminists have demonstrated how non-disabled women's participation in the world outside the home has been, and still is, more problematic than men's access to the public realm (Abel & Nelson, 1990; Finch, 1989; Gerson, 1985). Research indicates that it is considerably more difficult to gain full membership in society if a woman has a disability (Fine & Asch, 1988). Despite this, only a small number of authors have raised the issue of community participation of women and men with disabilities from a gender perspective. This small but fast growing international body of literature uses a feminist framework to analyse the disability field and, in particular, how gender influences the lives of men and women with disabilities (see for example Barron, 1997; Driedger, Feika & Batres, 1996; Fine and Asch, 1988; Hanna and Rogovsky, 1992; Johnson, 1998; Morris, 1991; Reinikainen, 1998; Traustadóttir, 1997a). Central to this work is the emphasis on gender as an important social dimension for all women and men—also those with a disability. Much of this literature has been devoted to identifying the barriers women with disabilities face in today's societies (Fine & Asch, 1988). It has been documented that they experience more difficulties than men with disabilities (and non-disabled women) in gaining access to many spheres of society such as education and employment, and their access to sexuality and intimacy is more limited than men's (Fine & Asch, 1988; Hannaford, 1985; Traustadóttir, 1997a). Unfortunately, this work has not had much impact on the current mainstream policies and practices in the field of developmental disabilities.

Figures from the United States show that women with disabilities receive considerably less education than men with disabilities (Asch & Fine, 1988; Bowe, 1984; Hanna and Rogovsky, 1991). In addition, there seems to be a difference in the educational experiences of men and women with disabilities. An example of this was found in a qualitative study of 30 women with developmental disabilities in Iceland conducted in 1996–1998 (Traustadóttir, 1997b; in press). Most of the women were in their twenties and thirties. They were all labelled as having a developmental disability ranging from mild to moderate and many of them had an additional disability. Despite the fact that students with disabilities in Iceland have had the legal right to an integrated education for over two decades, the majority of the women had attended segregated schools or classrooms for all, or most of, their education. Only about half of them continued their education after completing the ten year compulsory schooling. The programs offered at the high school level were gender stereotypical, reinforced the existing gender stereotypes, and did nothing to counteract the difficulties women with disabilities have had in gaining access to paid work. As a result, the majority of the 30 women had experienced great difficulties in gaining access to employment in the regular labor market.

These findings are consistent with studies of the employment difficulties facing women with disabilities in other countries. A number of studies have shown that women with disabilities fare significantly worse than men when it comes to employment (Bowe, 1984; Trupin, Sebesta, Yelin, & LaPlante, 1997; Hanna & Rogovsky, 1991; Russo & Jansen, 1988). The participation of women with disabilities in the labor market seems to be considerably more problematic than men's. In addition, if women with disabilities do get work they are more likely to have part time jobs while men with disabilities hold full time jobs. This seems to hold true for all types and levels of disabilities. In fact, some studies show that men with disabilities are almost twice as likely to have jobs than women with disabilities. Women with disabilities who are employed also receive considerably lower wages than their male counterparts. In a study of the relative importance of impairment and gender in predicting income of people with disabilities, Barnartt and Altman (1997) found that gender had more influence on wages than impairment. In addition to receiving lower wages tahn men, women with disabilities do not receive economic and social support to the same extent as men with disabilities. For example, in a recent US study, Baldwin (1997) analysed the gender differences in social security income programs (Social Security Disability Insurance: SSDI and Supplemental Security Income: SSI) and found that women received income from these sources at significantly lower levels than men did. These programs are intended to provide income for individuals who do not work. Not having access to this source of income to the same extent as men with disabilities, as well as having no or lower wages, points to a pattern of gender-based income discrimination. As a result, women with disabilities are likely to experience more difficulties than their male counterparts in surviving outside residential programs and participating in community life.

Most research on the employment of women with disabilities is based on information about women with physical disabilities. Only a handful of studies provide information about employment of women with developmental disabilities. These indicate that women with developmental disabilities are subject to the same employment barriers as women with other disabilities. A new initiative, supported employment, has been developed within the field of developmental disabilities to assist those with even the most severe disabilities to get and hold a job. This new initiative recognises the importance of productive work as a means to achieve social equality, financial independence, and access to everyday community life for all people with disabilities. Supported employment started in the United States but is now being developed in many other countries as well (see Moon, Inge, Wehman, Brooke, & Barcus (1990) for descriptions of such programs in the US). The initial goal of supported employment was to assist people with severe developmental disabilities who traditionally had experienced difficulties in gaining access to regular jobs. Supported employment was framed in the context of level of disability and did not take other issues, such as gender, into consideration. Despite the fact that women with developmental disabilities constitute a group that has traditionally had problems accessing the labor marked, supported employment ignored the specific barriers experienced by woman.

In the recent wealth of research and writing about supported employment little attention has been devoted to the employment difficulties faced by women. Only a handful of studies have reported gender differences in supported employment. These studies reported that men with developmental disabilities were more likely than women to be placed in jobs through supported employment programs and were more likely to retain their jobs than women. For example, in a study of a group of 186 individuals with developmental disabilities who had been placed in competitive jobs through supported employment programs, researchers found a "disproportionate representation of males (68% male go 32% female) in the population of placed consumers" (Kregel & Wehman, 1989: 265). The same trend was found by Hill et al. (1985) in a study of a group with the same disability. These studies indicate that the new approaches in the field of developmental disabilities retain the same pattern of gender discrimination as the older approaches.

The same employment discrimination was found in the qualitative study of women with developmental disabilities in Iceland (Traustadóttir, in press). The study revealed that men were considerably more likely than women to receive employment through the largest employment agency in the capital city, Reykjavík, which placed individuals with developmental disabilities in jobs in regular work places. In addition, women with developmental disabilities needed more education and training than men with disabilities in order to be considered to have adequate training to participate in the regular labor market.

The barriers to full participation of women with disabilities in community life are complex. One of these barriers has to do with abuse and violence. It is widely documented that women with disabilities are more likely than most other groups of women to experience abuse of various kinds: physical, emotional, and sexual (Asch & Fine, 1988; Sobsey & Doe, 1991; Sobsey, Wells, Lucardie, & Mansell, 1995). Instead of taking serious measures to make the community a safer place for women with disabilities, the most common attempt to prevent abuse and violence against them is to limit their access to various community places. Thus, family members' and service providers' fears of abuse can, and often do, result in limits to community participation of women with disabilities. In a study of institutional closure in Australia, Johnson (1998) provides a good example of this. The study focused on a group of twenty-one women with developmental disabilities and challenging behaviours who lived in a locked unit in a large institution and followed them through the process of deinstitutionalization. Johnson discusses how the women's sexuality sometimes was one of the determining factors in deciding their future after moving out of the institution. The possibility that the women could become vulnerable to sexual abuse in the community was feared by their families and could be the main reason for them being placed in another institution rather than in the community. Thus, in the process of deinstitutionalization, women and men with developmental disabilities are likely to be considered for different placements based on their gender which can result in a more restricted community participation of women with developmental disabilities than men.

There are many aspects of the lives and experiences of women with disabilities we do not know about. What we do know, however, is that disability programs often affect them differently than men with disabilities. The result seems to be that women with disabilities have, on the average, lower levels of community participation than men with the same disabilities. The current reforms toward full participation of people with disabilities in all aspects of community life have traditionally not taken into account issues of gender nor the double discrimination against women with disabilities. Most people in the field do not seem to be aware of how this double disadvantage results in more difficulties in community participation for women with disabilities. Policy and practices in the field have not been designed to meet the specific needs of women with disabilities, whether the needs relate to education, employment and income, or marriage childbearing, and parenting. Researchers, agencies, professionals, and policy makers need to be more sensitive to the specific barriers women with disabilities face when they attempt to become full participants in community life.

CHILDREN WITH DISABILITIES, THEIR FAMILIES, AND THE GENDERED DIVISION OF CARING

Since the beginning of the reform most countries have given priority to children with disabilities. These countries have made a commitment to keep children with disabilities in families and some have developed policies that ban institutionalization of children. As a result, increasing numbers of children with disabilities, including those with the most severe disabilities, are now living with their families.

Research directed towards families of children with disabilities has also been one of the distinguishing characteristics of the reform and there has been vigorous research in this area. This research has most commonly been characterized by an emphasis on the importance of families in the lives of these children (Farber, 1986; Gallagher & Vietze, 1986; Singer & Irvin, 1989). Much of this literature has attempted to determine the areas where families of children with disabilities need assistance in caring for their children at home and many authors advocate for more family support programs to assist families (Taylor, Racino, Knoll, & Lutfiyya, 1987). As a result, public policies directed toward families of children with disabilities have been one of the most visible parts of the community integration policies and practices, and family support services have emerged as an important component of the new community-based services.

While the growing interest in families of children with disabilities should be welcomed, a review of the research literature raises concerns due to the lack of critical examination of gender within these families. The vast majority of the literature which has informed both policies and practices directed toward families of children with disabilities has been based on a view of the "family" as a unit. The family, and sometimes "parents," are treated as the smallest unit of analysis and the differences in activities and experiences of individual family members have, for the most part, been ignored. These studies are routinely characterized by what Eichler (1988) refers to as "gender insensitivity." That is, they ignore gender as an important social dimension, thereby hiding the differences between mothers and fathers within the family, as well as differences within gender. The practice of treating the family as the unit of analysis and disregarding gender as an important aspect of family life has also served to hide from view the gendered organization of caring work in families. This is particularly interesting given the fact that studies focusing on families of children with disabilities living at home show that mothers have the main responsibilities for caring for the child within the family (Traustadóttir, 1995; Wickham-Searl, 1992).

When studying families, researchers usually collect information from mothers and the overwhelming majority of family studies within the disability field have focused on mothers. When writing up their findings, however, authors most often refer to the family's, or the parents' views and experiences, even if their findings are mainly, or solely, based upon information from the mothers. This has at least two consequences. First, even if mothers are overrepresented in research samples, the research reports hide the mothers and their experiences by referring to parents or families. Second, the underrepresentation of fathers leaves us without knowledge and understanding of the fathers' views and experiences.

Thus, instead of focusing on gender as an issue of inquiry, most disability family studies reflect the cultural stereotype of mothers as the "natural" caregivers and assume that women's primary orientation is toward family and motherhood (Bright & Wright, 1986; Munford, 1994; Traustadóttir, 1995). This both reflects and constructs how the disability field views, understands, and interprets the lives of mothers and fathers of children with disabilities, as well as the caring work within these families. We need a critical analysis of caring work in families of children with disabilities which challenges this traditional interpretation of families and draws upon a feminist critique of family life in examining the caring work of mothers who have children with disabilities.

Service providers seem to have different views and expectations of mothers and fathers. The mother, who plays a central role in the caring work, is typically also the main contact person for the service providers. While service providers and professionals do not see themselves as having authority over fathers and are reluctant to put demands on fathers, they are less reluctant to pressure the mothers. They routinely demand a certain level of co-operation and performance from the mother, and most of them see it as their duty to influence what she does with her child with a disability. This raises concerns about the way family support services influence and control the lives of mothers who have children with disabilities (Traustadóttir, 1991).

At least two of the rationales used in favor of family support policies are based on assumptions that are problematic for women. The first rationale is economic and asserts that family support services save money because they prevent costly out-of-home placements and may encourage families to take their children home from institutions and nursing homes (Taylor, Racino, Knoll, & Lutfiyya, 1987). This rationale is supported by cost studies of services. When researchers have compared the cost of residential placements and the cost of home care, they have found enormous savings when the care is provided in the family (Bradley, 1988; Governor's Planning Council on Developmental Disabilities, 1987). The second rationale is ideological. Family support services are seen as supporting traditional family values, and the main goal of many family support services is to support the family as a unit, keep families intact, and help families take care of their own. These two rationales have been used to convince policy makers and service providers to fund and provide family support services and are viewed as powerful arguments in favour of family policy directed toward families of children with disabilities (Taylor, Racino, Knoll, & Lutfiyya, 1987).

A critical examination of these two rationales raises serious concerns about the underlying assumptions about mothers of children with disabilities. The first concern is related to the cost savings of family support services. Why do these services save money? Given the gendered division of caring work in families, the consequence of this rationale places increased responsibility for caring on women and family support services save money because mothers provide much of the care needed by their children at no public cost.

The other concern relates to the idea of traditional family values. There are many different definitions of traditional family values and an appeal to these values without further clarification of what that means raises concern because, for many people, traditional family values bring to mind the culturally sanctified female role of caretaking and selfless giving. Traditional ideas and values about women's and men's roles within the family assign the responsibility for housework, child care, and other caring work to women, and women continue to perform large amounts of unpaid work in the family (Waring, 1988). These traditional values also assume that women's primary orientation is toward family and that they have little commitment to paid employment. Yet, the reality today is that the majority of women are trying to negotiate their caring work within the family with work outside the home (Baldwin & Glendinning, 1983; Berg, 1986; Abel & Nelson, 1990; Finch, 1989; Gerson, 1985). An uncritical emphasis on these two rationales may lead to some serious dilemmas or conflicts and we must ask if we are basing family support services on an outdated understanding of women's situation in today's societies. We should also consider to what extent current family policy assumes and depends on the substantial and consistent input of women's unpaid work in the home. Misguided family policies can jeopardise the possibilities of children with disabilities to participate in family and community life.

Policy makers and service providers need to become aware of the stereotypical assumptions underlying disability policies and practices. In particular, they need to recognize gender as a critical issue when policy and practices are formulated, instead of approaching families with a view that ignores gender, thereby reinforcing women's subordinate position in society.

Gender and Caring Work in the Human Services

Women constitute the great majority of workers within disability services. Despite this, limited attention has been directed toward the women who work in the service system and carry out the reform. Those who have written about the community-based services, personnel preparation, and the new approaches of the reform rarely mention the fact that the majority of the workers are women.

The reason for this invisibility of the women who bear the brunt of the daily work of the reform seems to derive from the power of the stereotype of women as caregivers. Women are seen as "natural" caregivers and it seems to be taken for granted that women occupy caregiving work within the human services as well as in other spheres of life (Abel & Nelson, 1990). Instead of taking for granted that the vast majority of workers in the field of developmental disabilities are women, we need to explore why women constitute most of those who work in the field. We need to analyse the processes by which women are recruited for caregiving for people with disabilities and examine the work of facilitating the acceptance and inclusion of people with disabilities in classrooms, work places, and other community places, and explore what this "inclusion work" has in common with women's traditional caregiving in families and communities.

We need to bring into view women's work of facilitating acceptance and inclusion of people with disabilities and supporting them to become a part of community life. Much of what women do in this context consists of activities we usually do not label as "work." Yet, many of these activities are similar to the caring work women have traditionally performed within their families and communities when they facilitate interactions between people, make them comfortable with each other, and bring people together in a social group (Traustadóttir, 1992). Caregiving is often described as an essential activity (Abel & Nelson, 1990; DeVault, 1991). The social fabric relies on the daily caring work of nurturing, maintaining, and sustaining life. The physical tasks and relational work performed by women human service workers in order to include people with disabilities in community life is also essential. It enables people with disabilities to interact with other people and participate in day-to-day activities alongside nondisabled community members. Without the efforts of these women many people with disabilities would not be part of families, classrooms, work places, churches, neighbourhoods, and so on (Traustadóttir & Taylor, 1998). The women who work in the human service system have a great deal of influence on the outcome of the current reform efforts in the field. There has, however, not been much attention on the women who work with people with disabilities. The reform seems to assume and depend upon these women, but does not often mention them.

The new community-based services established to carry out the reform have experienced difficulties in achieving community participation of people with disabilities. It has been particularly problematic for these programs to facilitate connections between people with disabilities and other community members. These problems in community services have led to a call for a shift in service delivery towards increased emphasis on relationships with nondisabled people. It has been particularly problematic for these programs to facilitate connections between people with disabilities and other community members. Connections are seen as "natural" community supports. The critics suggest radical changes in current services and have outlined an alternative to the traditional approach in community programs. The new approaches should start with the person and an examination of his or her social networks and informal community supports. Then design formal support interventions which build on and strengthen natural networks in the community (Smull & Bellamy, 1991; Taylor, Bogdan, & Racino, 1991).

This new emphasis has led to a growing interest and appreciation of the importance of informal supports and personal relationships in the lives of children and adults with disabilities (Amado, 1993; Beach Center on Families and Disability, 1997; Forest, 1989; Hutchison, 1990; Lutfiyya, 1991; Taylor & Bogdan, 1989; Taylor, Bogdan, & Lutfiyya, 1995). The criticism of community-based programs has also led to a growing interest in exploring how to integrate formal supports (provided through services agencies and programs), and informal supports in the community (based on personal ties and social relationships) (Bulmer, 1987).

These new approaches in service delivery have been accompanied by a call for a new role for human service workers; especially those who work directly with people with disabilities (Gardner & Chapman, 1992; Kaiser & McWhorter, 1990). For example, Knoll & Ford (1987) argue that in order to provide adults with severe disabilities the necessary support to become actively involved in their home and communities, we need to reconceptualize direct-care workers as facilitators of relationships. The most important part of the new role of direct care staff should be to work toward natural supports through assisting people with severe disabilities to establish nonpaid relationships with regular community members (as opposed to relationships with workers who are paid to be with the person), as well as helping people maintain existing relationships with family and friends.

Implied is the belief that such personal relationships will serve as a basis for the supports necessary for people with disabilities to participate fully in community life. The belief that true inclusion of people with disabilities can only be achieved through supportive personal relationships with nondisabled people is beginning to influence policies and practices in the field of developmental disabilities. For example, fieldwork in human service organizations in the United States has shown that the workers in the field, especially those who worked in direct services (and the vast majority of these people are women), were being encouraged to establish personal relationships with the people with disabilities they worked with (Traustadóttir, 1992). The same study found that, within some service agencies, it had become a measurement of a "good worker" whether she had made such a personal commitment or not. As a result, an increasing number of women had made commitments to people with disabilities that went far beyond the formal requirements of their jobs.

The same study showed that a new language had emerged to describe these workers and what they did: they were "committed and involved." The language of "commitment and involvement" had not only been adopted by those who worked within the field of developmental disabilities, it was also used within the institutions that trained professionals for the field. For example, during the process of soliciting nominations of female workers and friends to participate in the study, many of the people used this language, including administrators, professionals, and college professors. The women who were nominated for the study and described as "very committed and involved" all had established a friendship with a person with a disability, which was the main reason for describing them in this way. Often there was no mention of these women's performance in other areas. The language of "committed and involved" had become so widespread that it had come to be commonly understood to mean "committed to people with disabilities" and "involved with people with disabilities in a personal relationship." Sometimes it even seemed as a test of people's "political correctness" whether they had a friend with a disability. Personal involvement and commitment had become the most important qualities professionals and para-professionals in the field of developmental disabilities could have, at least in those service agencies that considered themselves to be progressive (Traustadóttir, 1992). This is in sharp contrast to the old language of "professional distance" and "impartial treatment" that used to be considered among the highest professional qualities.

From the time they are little girls, women are trained to be nurturing, caring, and attuned to the needs of others (Gilligan, 1982). This makes women particularly susceptible for arguments that encourage them to make personal commitments to people in need (Traustadóttir, 1993). In addition, at the heart of many women's work with people with disabilities is the desire to change the injustices experienced by people with disabilities and their work is often performed in the context of a vision of a world where people with disabilities are welcomed, loved, and included. All of this makes women who work in human services easy targets for the pressure to make an even stronger commitment and become even more involved (Traustadóttir, 1992).

In a study of female humans service workers in the US, Traustadóttir and Taylor (1998) found strong indications that current disability policies have had considerable impact on the women who work in the human services. The women who participated in the study had made personal commitments to people with disabilities that far exceeded the formal requirements of their jobs. This is one more example of the continuing process of the recruitment of women to care for others, a process that starts in childhood and continues throughout women's adult lives.

This pressure on women to make a personal commitment to at least one person with a disability, and become involved in the life of that person beyond what is required by their job, makes it hard for women to place limits on their working hours. This also makes it hard for women to distinguish between what is "work" (paid human service work) and what is "personal commitment" (unpaid caring work based on a personal relationship). As a result of these fluid boundaries of women's human service work, many of them experience a conflict in terms of the various demands on their time and caring work. They are torn between demands from their families, on the one hand, and demands on their time from their human service work and commitments, on the other. The difficulties women have in placing limits on their human service work brings economic benefits to the service system. The caring work these women perform in the name of personal commitment is no longer defined as "work" if it is done outside their working hours. Instead, it is defined as "friendship" or "commitment."

It appears as if current disability policies are moving the boundaries of women's responsibilities within the human services in a way that creates pressures on women to increase the work they perform without being compensated. It seems as though it is no longer enough for women to perform their job well. If they want to earn the highest praise in the field—the praise of being "committed and involved"—they have to go beyond the formal job requirements and make a personal commitment to become involved in the lives of people with disabilities outside their paid working hours.

The current trend in the field has, at least partly, resulted in the recruitment of women to perform significant amounts of caring work for people with disabilities without being paid for it. In times of declining resources for human services, this transfer of paid work over to friendship is economically convenient. When accompanied by suggestions that "natural support" should replace some of, or most of, publicly funded services, current disability policies may place women in a position to be exploited.

The field of developmental disabilities needs to take a serious look at some of the fundamental assumptions behind policy and practices. The field can no longer ignore the important contributions women have made, and continue to make, to the field. Without women's competent and skillful work of attending to the needs of others and bringing people together in a social context, current reforms would not have been possible. Women's contributions need to be recognized, made visible, and justly compensated. These contributions are essential for the participation of people with disabilities in community life. This work should be shared more equally and be better supported by society's institutions so that women are not expected to provide the work necessary to achieve acceptance and inclusion of people with disabilities at the expense of equity.

Conclusion

Current disability reform has been carried out without much conscious awareness or understanding of how issues of gender influence the lives of people with disabilities. There is also a curious lack of recognizing the important contributions women have made to the reform. Despite the fact that women perform the vast majority of the day-to-day work of the reform, their contributions remain largely unnoticed and invisible. At the same time, women are being recruited to perform increasing amounts of caring work for people with disabilities, without being paid for it. This suggests a conflict between the disability reform and women's concerns and the danger of exploiting women in the efforts to liberate people with disabilities. We need to find ways of implementing the reform that benefits both women caregivers and people with disabilities. There is also a need to understand how disability programs affect the lives of women and men with disabilities in different ways. Policy makers and service providers need to become aware of the stereotypical and gendered assumptions underlying most disability policies and practices. In particular, they need to recognize gender as a critical issue when policies and practices are formulated, instead of approaching disability issues with a view that ignores gender and thereby reinforces women's subordinate position in society. If the field of developmental disabilities continues to ignore gender as a fundamental issue when policies and practices are formulated, these will remain fundamentally flawed and continue to hinder the full participation of people with disabilities in everyday community life.

References

Abel, E. K. & Nelson, M. K. (1990) (Eds.). Circles of care: *Work and identity in women's lives.* Albany, NY: State University of New York Press.

Amado, A. K. (Ed.)(1993). *Friendships and community connections between people with and without disabilities.* Baltimore: Paul H. Brookes.

Asch, A. & Fine, M. (1988). *Introduction: Beyond pedestals.* In M. Fine & A. Asch (Eds.), *Women with disabilities: Essays in psychology, culture, and politics* (pp. 1-37). Philadelphia: Temple University Press.

Baldwin, M. L. (1997). *Gender differences in social security disability decisions.* Journal of Disability Policy Studies, Special Issue on Gender and Disability Policy,8(1&2), pp. 25-50.

Baldwin, S., & Glendinning, C. (1983). Employment, women and their disabled children. In J. Finch & D. Groves (Eds.), A labour of love: Women, work and caring (pp. 53-71). London: Routledge & Kegan Paul.

Barnartt, S. N., & Altman, B. M. (1997). *Predictors of wages: Comparisons by gender and type of impairment.* Journal of Disability Policy Studies, Special Issue on Gender and Disability Policy, 8(1&2), pp. 51-74.

Barron, K. (1997). *Disability and gender: Autonomy as an indication of adulthood.* Uppsala: Uppsala University

Beach Center on Families and Disability (1997). *Amistad: Stories of Hispanic children with disabilties and their friendships.* Lawrence, Kansas: Author.

Berg, B. J. (1986). *The crisis of the working mother: Resolving the conflict between family and work.* New York: Summit Books

Bérubé, M. (1996). *Life as we know it: A father, a family, and an exceptional child. New York:* Pantheon Books.

Bowe, F. (1984). *Disabled women in America: A statistical report drawn from census data.* Washington, DC: President's Committee on Employment of the Handicapped.

Bradley, V. J. (1988). *The Medical Family and Community Quality Service Act: How does it address research findings, quality assurance, and family support?* A statement prepared for US Senate Finance Committee, United State Senate. Washington, DC.

Bradley, V. J., Ashbaugh, J. W., & Blaney, B. C. (Eds.) (1994) *Creating individual supports for people with developmental disabilities: A mandate for change at many levels.* Baltimore: Paul H. Brookes.

Bright, R.W. & Wright, J.M.C. (1986). *Community-based services: The impact on mothers of children with disabilities.* Australian and New Zealand Journal of Developmental Disabilities, 12(4), 223-228.

Brown, H. & Smith, H. (1992). *Assertion not assimilation: A feminist perspective on the normalisation principle.* In H. Brown & H. Smith (Eds.). Normalisation: A reader for the nineties. London: Travistock/Routledge.

Bulmer, M. (1987). *The social basis of community care.* London: Allen & Unwin.

DeVault, M. (1991). *Feeding the family: The social organization of caring as gendered work.* Chicago: University of Chicago Press.

Driedger, D., Feika, I., & Batres, E. G. (Eds.) (1996). *Across borders: Women with disabilities working together.* Charlottetown, PEI: gynergy books.

Eichler, M. (1988). Nonsexist research methods. Boston: Unwin.

Fadiman, A. (1997). *The spirit catches you and you fall down: A Hmong child, her American doctors, and the collision of two cultures.* New York: Farrar, Straus and Giroux.

Farber, B. (1986). *Historical contexts of research on families with mentally retarded members.* In I.J. Gallagher & P.M. Vietze, (Eds.). Families of handicapped persons: Research, programs, and policy issues (pp. 3-23). Baltimore: Paul H. Brookes.

Fine, M. and Asch., A. (Eds.)(1988). *Women with disabilities: Essays in psychology, culture and politics.* Philadelphia: Temple University Press

Finch, J. (1989). *Family obligations and social change.* Cambridge: Policy Press.

Forest, M. (1989). *It's about relationships.* Toronto: Frontier College Press.

Gallagher, J. J., & Vietze, P. M. (Eds.)(1986*). Families of handicapped persons: Research, programs, and policy issues.* Baltimore: Paul H. Brookes.

Gardener, J., & Champman, M. S. (1992). *Developing staff competencies for supporting people with developmental disabilities: An orientation handbook* (2nd ed.). Baltimore: Paul H. Brookes.

Gerson, K. (1985). *Hard choices: How women decide about work, career, and motherhood.* Berkeley: University of California Press.

Gilligan, C. (1982). *In a different voice: Psychological theory and women's development.* Cambridge, MA: Harvard University Press.

Governor's Planning Council on Developmental Disabilities (1987). *Supporting family care of persons who are developmentally disabled:* Family support/cash subsidy programs. Springfield, IL: Author

Hanna, W. I., & Rogovsky, E. (1991). *Women with disabilities: Two handicaps plus. Disability, Handicap & Society*, 6(1), 49-63

Hanna, W. I., & Rogovsky, E. (1992). *On the situation of African American women with physical disabilities.* Journal of Applied Rehabilitation Counselling, 23(4), 39-45

Hannaford, S. (1985). *Living outside inside: A disabled woman's experience: Towards a social and political perspective.* Berkeley: Canterbury Press.

Harry, B. (1992). *Cultural diversity, families, and the special education system: Communication and empowerment.* New York: Teachers College Press.

Hayden, M. F. & Abery, B. (Eds.)(1994). *Challenges for a service system in transition: Ensuring quality experiences for persons with developmental disabilities.* Baltimore: Paul H. Brookes.

Hill, J.W., Hill, M., Wehman, P., Banks, P. D., Pendleton, P., & Britt, C. (1985). *Demographic analysis related to successful job retention for competitively employed persons who are mentally retarded.* In P. Wehman & J.W. Hill (Eds.), *Competitive employment for persons with mental retardation: From research to practice* (Vol. I). Richmond: Rehabilitation Research and Training Center, Virginia Commonwealth University.

Hutchison, P. (1990). *Making friends: Developing relationships between people with a disability and other members of the community.* Toronto: G. Allan Roeher Institute.

Johnson, K. (1998). *Deinstitutionalising women: An ethnographic study of institutional closure.* Melbourne: Cambridge University Press.

Kaiser, A. P., & McWhorter, C. M. (1990). *Preparing personnel to work with persons with severe disabilities.* Baltimore: Paul H. Brookes.

Kalyanpur, M., & Rao, S. (1991). *Empowering low-income black families of handicapped children.* American Journal of Orthopsychiatry, 61(4), 523-532.

Keith, L. (1994). *Mustn't grumble: Writings by disabled women.* New York: The New Press.

Knoll, J., & Ford, A. (1987). *Beyond caregiving: A reconceptualization of the role of the residential service provider.* In S. J. Taylor, D. Biklen, & J. Knoll (Eds.), Community integration for people with severe disabilities (pp. 129-146). New York: Teachers College Press.

Kregel, J. & Wehman, P. (1989). *An analysis of the employment outcomes of young adults with mental retardation.* In P. Wehman & J. Kregel (Eds.) *Supported employment for persons with disabilities: Focus on excellence.* New York: Human Sciences Press.

Lorber, J. & Farrell, S.A. (1991). *The social construction of gender.* Newbury Park, CA: Sage.

Lynch, E. W., & Hanson, M. J. (1992). *Developing cross-cultural competence: A guide for working with young children and their families.* Baltimore: Paul H. Brookes.

Lutfiyya, Z. M. (1991). *"A feeling of being connected": Friendships between people with and without learning difficulties.* Disability, Handicap & Society, 6(3), 233-245.

Moon, M. S., Inge, K. J., Wehman, P., Brooke, V., & Barcus, J. M. (1990). *Helping persons with severe mental retardation get and keep employment: Supported employment issues and strategies.* Baltimore: Paul H. Brookes.

Morris, J. (1991). *Pride against prejudice: Transforming attitudes to disability.* Philadelphia: New Society Publishers.

Morris, J. (1996)(Ed.). *Encounters with strangers: Feminism and disability.* London: The Women's Press.

Munford, R. (1994). *Caregiving: A shared commitment.* In K. Ballard (Ed.) Disability, family, whanau and society (pp 265-292), Palmerson North: Dunmore Press.

O'Connor, S. (1992). *"I'm not an Indian anymore": The challenge of providing culturally sensitive services to American Indians.* In J. A. Racino, P. Walker, S. O'Connor, & S. J. Taylor (Eds.), *Housing, support, and community: Choices and strategies for adults with disabilities.* Baltimore: Paul H. Brookes.

O'Connor, S. (1993). *Multiculturalism and disability: A collection of resources and issues.* Syracuse, NY: Center on Human Policy, Syracuse University.

Reinikainen, M. R. (1998, August). *The bodies of disabled women and men: Are they equal?* A paper presented at the Summer School, University of Jyväskylä, Finland.

Richardson, L. & Taylor, L. (Eds.)(1993). *Feminist frontiers III.* New York: McGraw-Hill.

Russo, N. F. & Jansen, M. A. (1988). *Women, work and disability: Opportunities and challenges.* In M. Fine & A. Asch (Eds.) *Women with disabilities: Essays in psychology, culture, and politics* (pp. 229-244). Philadelphia, PA: Temple University Press.

Sandvin, J. T. (1993). *Mot normalt? Omsorgsideologier i forandring (Toward the normal? Changing caring ideologies)*. Oslo: Kommuneforlaget.

Sandvin, J.T., Söder, M., Lichtwarck, W., & Magnussen, (1998). *Normaliseringsarbeid og ambivalens: Bofelleskap som ormsorgsarena (Normalizationwork and ambivalence: Residential services as a sphere of caring)*. Oslo: Universitetsforlaget.

Scheerenberger, R. C. (1983). *A history of mental retardation*. Baltimore: Paul H. Brookes.

Scheerenberger, R. C. (1987). *A history of mental retardation: A quarter century of promise*. Baltimore: Paul H. Brookes.

Singer, G. H. S., & Irvin, L. K. (Eds.). (1989). *Support for caregiving families: Enabling positive adaptation to disability*. Baltimore: Paul H. Brookes.

Smull, M. W., & Bellamy, G. T. (1991). *Community services for adults with disabilities: Policy challenges in the emerging support paradigm*. In L. Meyer, C. Peck, & L. Brown (Eds.), Critical issues in the lives of people with severe disabilities (pp. 527-536). Baltimore: Paul H. Brookes.

Traustadóttir, R. (1995). *A mother's work is never done: Constructing a "normal" family life*. In S. J. Taylor, R. Bogdan, & Z. M. Lutfiyya (Eds.). The variety of community experience: Qualitative studies of family and community life, (pp. 47-65). Baltimore: Paul H. Brookes.

Traustadóttir, R. (1997a). *Women with disabilities: Issues, resources, connections*. Updated by Perri Harris. Syracuse, NY: Center on Human Policy, Syracuse University.

Traustadóttir, R. (1997b). *Kvenleiki og fötlun (Womanliness and disability.)* In Helga Kress & Rannveig Traustadóttir (Eds.), Íslenskar kvennarannsóknir (Icelandic women's studies). Reykjavík: Háskóli Íslands, Rannsóknastofa í kvennafræ?um.

Traustadóttir, R. (in press). *Líka fyrir fatla?ar konur? Margbreytileiki og minnihlutahópar í íslensku samfélagi (What about women with disabilities? Multiculturalism and minority groups in Icelandic society)*. In F.H. Jónsson (Ed.) Rannsóknir í félagsvísindum (Research in Social Sciences) Reykjavík: Félagsvísindastofnun Háskóla Íslands og Háskólaútgáfan.

Traustadóttir, R., Shoultz, B., & Lutfiyya, Z. M. (1994). *Community integration: A multicultural perspective*. In M. F. Hayden & B. Abery (Eds.), Challenges for a service system in transition: Ensuring quality experiences for persons with developmental disabilities (pp. 405-426). Baltimore: Paul H. Brookes.

Traustadóttir, R. & Taylor, S. J. (1998). *Invisible women, invisible work: Women's caring work in developmental disability services*. In S. J. Taylor & R. Bogdan, Introduction to qualitative research methods.: A guidebook and resource, 3rd revised edition (pp. 205-220). New York: John Wiley.

Tøssebro, J., Gustavsson, A., & Dyredal, B. (Eds.). (1996). *Intellectual disabilities in the Nordic welfare states: Policies and everyday life*. Kristiansand: Norwegian Academic Press.

Waring, M. (1988). *If women counted: A new feminist economics*. New York: HarperSan Francisco.

Wickham-Searl, P. (1992). *Careers in caring: Mothers of children with disabilities*. Disability, Handicap and Society, 7(1), 5-18.

Wilson, P. G., O'Reilly, M. F., & Rusch, F. R. (1991). *Analysis of minority-status supported employees in relation to placement approach and selected outcomes*. Mental Retardation, 29(6), 329-333.

Sobsey, D. & Doe, T. (1991). *Patterns of sexual abuse and assault*. Sexuality and Disability, 9(3), 243-260.

Sobsey, D., Wells, D., Lucardie, R., & Mansell, S. (1995). *Violence and disability: An annotated bibliography* Baltimore: Paul H. Brookes.

Taylor, S. J., & Bogdan, R. (1989). *On accepting relationships between people with mental retardation and nondisabled people: Towards an understanding of acceptance*. Disability, Handicap & Socciety, 4(1), 21-36.

Taylor, S. J., Biklen, D., & Knoll, J. (Eds.)(1987). *Community integration for people with severe disabilities*. New York: Teacher College Press.

Taylor, S. J., Bogdan, R., & Lutfiyya, Z. M. (Eds.)(1995). *The variety of community experience: Qualitative studies of family and community life*. Baltimore: Paul H. Brookes

Taylor, S. J., Bogdan, R., & Racino, J. A. (Eds.). (1991). *Life in the community: Case studies of organizations supporting people with disabilities*. Baltimore: Paul H. Brookes.

Taylor, S. J., Racino, J. A., Knoll, J. A., & Lutfiyya, Z. M. (1987). *The nonrestrictive environment: On community integration for people with the most severe disabilities.* Syracuse, NY: Human Policy Press.

Tong, R.P. (1998). *Feminist thought (2nd Ed.)* Boulder, CO: Westview Press.

Trupin, L, Sebesta, D. S., Yelin, E., and LaPlante, M P. (1997). *Trends in the labor force participation among persons with disabilities,* 1983-1994. Disability Statistics Report (10). Washington, DC: US Department of Education, National Institute on Disability and Rehabilitation Research.

Traustadóttir, R. (1991). *Mothers who care: Gender, disability, and family life. Journal of Family Issues, Special Issue on Gender and Unpaid Work,* 12(2).

Traustadóttir, R. (1992). *Disability reform and the role of women: Community inclusion and caring work.* Syracuse, NY: Syracuse University. Unpublished Ph.D. dissertation.

Traustadóttir, R. (1993). *The gendered context of friendship. In A. N. Amado (Ed.), Friendships and community connections between people with and without disabilities,* (pp. 109-27). Baltimore: Paul H. Brookes.

Traustadóttir, R. (1995). *A mother's work is never done: Constructing a "normal" family life.* In S. J. Taylor, R. Bogdan, & Z. M. Lutfiyya (Eds.). *The variety of community experience: Qualitative studies of family and community life,* (pp. 47-65). Baltimore: Paul H. Brookes.

Traustadóttir, R. (1997a). *Women with disabilities: Issues, resources, connections.* Updated by Perri Harris. Syracuse, NY: Center on Human Policy, Syracuse University.

Traustadóttir, R. (1997b). *Kvenleiki og fötlun (Womanliness and disability.) In Helga Kress & Rannveig Traustadóttir (Eds.), Íslenskar kvennarannsóknir (Icelandic women's studies).* Reykjavík: Háskóli Íslands, Rannsóknastofa í kvennafræ?um.

Traustadóttir, R. (in press). *Líka fyrir fatla?ar konur? Margbreytileiki og minnihlutahópar í íslensku samfélagi (What about women with disabilities? Multiculturalism and minority groups in Icelandic society). In F.H. Jónsson (Ed.) Rannsóknir í félgasvísindum* (Research in Social Sciences) Reykjavík: Félagsvísindastofnun Háskóla Íslands og Háskólaútgáfan.

Traustadóttir, R., Shoultz, B., & Lutfiyya, Z. M. (1994). *Community integration: A multicultural perspective.* In M. F. Hayden & B. Abery (Eds.), *Challenges for a service system in transition: Ensuring quality experiences for persons with developmental disabilities* (pp. 405-426). Baltimore: Paul H. Brookes.

Traustadóttir, R. & Taylor, S. J. (1998). *Invisible women, invisible work: Women's caring work in developmental disability services.* In S. J. Taylor & R. Bogdan, Introduction to qualitative research methods.: A guidebook and resource, 3rd revised edition (pp. 205-220). New York: John Wiley.

Tøssebro, J., Gustavsson, A., & Dyredal, B. (Eds.). (1996). *Intellectual disabilities in the Nordic welfare states: Policies and everyday life.* Kristiansand: Norwegian Academic Press.

Waring, M. (1988). *If women counted: A new feminist economics.* New York: HarperSan Francisco.

Wickham-Searl, P. (1992). *Careers in caring: Mothers of children with disabilities.* Disability, Handicap and Society, 7(1), 5-18.

Wilson, P. G., O'Reilly, M. F., & Rusch, F. R. (1991). *Analysis of minority-status supported employees in relation to placement approach and selected outcomes. Mental Retardation,* 29(6), 329-333.

23

In Her Own Home
The Experiences of Catherine Schaefer

Zana Marie Lutfiyya
Department of Educational Administration, Foundations & Psychology
Faculty of Education, University of Manitoba

In 1986, Catherine Schaefer moved from her parents' home to her own place. She lives on the main floor of a spacious house on a street flanked with elms and oaks so tall they form a canopy overhead. There is a park across the street from her home. Like many of the houses in this neighbourhood, there are two additional apartments on the second and third floors.

Catherine leads an active life: she swims several times a week, visits her family and friends and has them over in turn. She sees her parents frequently and spends major holidays at her mother's home. Her two younger brothers both live out of town, and she is thrilled to see them when they visit.

The story of Catherine and her family is well documented elsewhere (Schaefer 1978, 1982, 1999) and will not be repeated here. Catherine needs extensive support in all areas of her life. This is provided through three community organizations: Prairie Housing Co-op, a not-for-profit housing co-operative, maintains her home; l'Avenir, a support co-operative, insures that Cath is able to live in her own home; and a third agency assists her to get out and about during the week. Family and friends also help to insure that Cath's needs are met and that her life is good. In so many ways, Cath's life isn't unusual. What is unusual is that a person with extensive physical and cognitive disabilities leads such an ordinary life, a life that many of us would simply take for granted. While Cath's life seems so outwardly typical, it is the direct result of an incredible amount of sustained effort on the part of a number of individuals. In this brief chapter, I will discuss some of the critical issues faced and lessons learned by those involved in this effort. In preparing this chapter, I had the opportunity to talk with Nicola Schaefer, Cath's mother, and two of Cath's first cousins, Paul and Sara. I also spoke with Darlene Stevens, a longtime family friend. Darlene was the first person to live with Catherine when she moved into her own home. I thank all these people for their time and consideration.

A large part of the effort to assist Catherine has to do with organization and organizations. The house has to be maintained, people to support Catherine must be identified, hired and trained. Communication among people and agencies is imperative to make sure that things run smoothly. While having three organizations involved is at times confusing, there are some benefits. First, Cath's housing is separated from her needs for assistance and support. Her supports are not tied to her place of residence. This means that she enjoys a measure of control over her home that many people living in group homes or other facilities do not enjoy.

Catherine receives assistance from l'Avenir, another co-operative. There is little bureaucracy within this agency; the focus is on members like Catherine. Founded by parents, l'Avenir boasts a high level of family involvement. Family members are consulted regularly as they help to interpret Catherine's needs. These relatively small organizations allow for a high degree of participation on the part of the people receiving support and their families in decision-making and planning. Having an organization also means that individuals and/or their families are not alone when they negotiate for funding and other supports from the provincial government.

Ensuring that Catherine enjoys a good life involves a number of critical issues. These include the control of the household, the actual provision of supports to Catherine and the ultimate question of safeguards.

Whose Home Is It Anyway?

Until early 1999, Catherine received support from a succession of live-in caregivers. These individuals typically stayed between one and two and a half years. This meant that a succession of people — arriving in different combinations of families with children, couples and single people — were living in the same apartment as Catherine, or in one of the other two apartments in the house. On a couple of occasions, Cath and her primary caregiver were joined by a friend of Cath's who shared her home as a roommate, but who did not provide any *paid* assistance or support to Cath, just friendship.

For almost fifteen years, and across several generations of support people, Cath shared her home with her primary paid caregiver. None of these individuals maintained another home, which meant that for a time, Cath's home was also their home. Although there was an awareness by the staff that they were living in Cath's home, they also needed the sense of belonging and comfort associated with living in one's own place. Caregivers tried to make themselves comfortable while also respecting Cath's preferences. However, home decor and furnishings changed as different people moved in and out. Household routines and the types of meals prepared varied, as did some of Cath's activities. Even Catherine's style of clothing tended to reflect the taste of her current primary caregiver.

In addition, people who visited the household changed when the caregivers changed. Some people remain constant, of course, like Cath's family and a small circle of friends. But each primary caregiver also invited new people over to visit. This practice both expanded Cath's world and curtailed it. She has met numerous people whom she might not otherwise have known. She has received invitations to all sorts of events and activities through the individuals who have provided support to her. As Cath does not talk, her friends and family must make arrangements to see her through the caregiver. In this way, the caregiver acts as a de facto gatekeeper to anyone who wishes to see Cath. The staff are often needed to drive Cath in her adapted van when she goes out and are again 'on duty' when friends and family come to visit. In many ways, Cath's domestic world often becomes that of her primary caregiver. (To a certain extent, the opposite happens - a few of us who met the Schaefers through taking care of Cath remain family friends years later).

Nicola talks about the need for Cath to have her own circle of friends, and the chance to pursue her own interests. But many of the people in Cath's life are there because they met Cath through Nicola, or they remain connected because Nicola provides the constant and consistent facilitation others need to keep in touch with Catherine. Nicola noted, "I'd love to eliminate myself from this...Cath needs to develop her own friends."

It is Nicola's belief that one of the main reasons for staff turnover is this dilemma about 'home'. While staff appreciate the paramount need for Cath's home to be truly her own, they are in effect homeless while living with her. Thinking about this, Nicola and others involved in supporting Cath came to the conclusion that they should try shift staffing. This began in 1999. The key support person meets Cath when she comes home in the afternoon, and spends the evening with her, but does not live in the house, nor does she sleep over. Another woman lives in/sleeps over and helps Cath out in the mornings. Care has been taken to make sure that the support staff are few and consistent. Nicola is also looking at co-housing as another option. In this scenario, Cath and several others (with and without disabilities) would each live in their own homes in a larger building or complex. Common areas for eating and socializing would insure interaction among neighbours on a daily basis. In this model, the people who support Cath could live in the co-housing complex or a different location altogether.

SUPPORTS

As Catherine needs assistance virtually all the time, she must be with someone who is willing and able to provide it. A delicate negotiation about who will do what must take place between Cath's paid caregivers and those who want to spend time with her. Until she moved out of her parents' home, her mother was the person who provided this assistance. Once she moved into her own home, Cath had to rely upon staff for this help. The exception to this is when Cath stays at her mother's house for a few days at a time, as she does at Christmas. Catherine's friends will often provide assistance when they get together (i.e, helping her eat at meals). But for the most part, Cath is surrounded by staff who drive her, push her wheelchair, help her eat and take part in a variety of other activities. Sometimes friends feel that a staff person is 'hovering' and almost interfering with their time with Cath, while others feel that the staff do not provide her with enough assistance. The negotiating begins all over again when staff change.

What does this mean? Those close to Catherine recognize that what goes on around her has impact on her. In some measure she mirrors the general atmosphere and disposition of those around her. When things are going well for staff and the others in her life, it is easier for Cath to be cheerful and healthy. During less sunny times, Cath may react by withdrawing, and not eating and drinking.

Nicola has another concern about the people who support Catherine. As she explained,

> Cath is 38 now, and I don't want to see her at the age of fifty surrounded only by 21 year olds. She needs to have people of all ages around her, including her peers.

While part of her concern may be addressed by having a variety of people in Cath's network of friends, there are implications here for who is chosen as paid support people. Nicola, who is involved in this process along with a staff person from l'Avenir, looks for a combination of support people who represent different ages and life experiences.

SAFEGUARDS

Parents naturally wonder and worry about what will happen to their children when they are no longer able to monitor their circumstances and to protect them. When asked about the issue of safeguarding Catherine, Nicola answered as many parents do. She talked about the importance of having many people involved in Catherine's life, a constant flow of people in and out of her home, people, paid or not, who will speak up if something is amiss. Nicola also believes it is important for the people around Catherine to know more than her likes and dislikes, more than the background information that appears in agency file folders. They need to know Cath's life story, the things that she has done, that she is able to do, in other words, who she is. This history can then be passed on in several ways. Photo albums and scrapbooks are reminders of important trips and other events. Mementos and gifts in Cath's home are indicators of the place that she has in the lives of others. Most important are family and friends, people with whom Cath has long term ties, people who know her and her history and pass it on to others.

While there are a number of individuals who do play this role, for the time being, it is Nicola who remains the ultimate safeguard for Catherine. She sees Catherine frequently and pays attention to what is happening in Cath's life. She is an active member of the l'Avenir board. She is acutely aware of the need to trust Cath to others while remaining concerned about her vulnerability. As she says, "... you can try to build in safeguards, but Cath is intensely vulnerable and can't speak for herself." In reviewing the ways in which Catherine remains at the mercy of others, she concludes, "This is called the dignity of risk. This is a great concept ... until it applies to Catherine!"

References

Schaefer, N. (1978). *Does she know she's there?* Toronto: Fitzhenry & Whiteside.

Schaefer, N. (1982). *Does she know she's there? Updated edition.* Toronto: Fitzhenry & Whiteside.

Schaefer, N. (1999). *Does she know she's there? 20th anniversary edition.* Toronto: Fitzhenry & Whiteside.

SECTION VI

Conclusion

24

Impatience, Mountains and the Moon

Gerald Provencal

> To fulfill the dreams of one's youth; that is the best that can happen to a man. No worldly success can take the place of that.
>
> *Willa Cather*

It was early in the El Nino summer of 1998 and my garden began to bloom like I was living in Georgia not Michigan when a friend asked me to write a piece for a tribute to Gunnar Dybwad. While I agreed and flushed with excitement, the invitation caught me at an awkward time. I was experiencing another mid-life crisis and this one was the most stubborn of all. First, it no longer could be seriously considered "mid" and, this time, I was more unsure about how to break the spell and move on. I was confident that a way would eventually clear yet, frankly, I felt more muddled about my career than at any time since freshman year.

My feelings were to a great extent bound to undeniable aging and its companion, the inevitable questioning and discounting of accomplishments by those in the next wave": the young Turks. Energetic, privileged, technologically gifted advocates and professional kids had, it seemed to me, all but taken over the part of human services work that once was the property of my friends and myself. More and more it seemed that they knew things that I had no clue about. They used jargon and acronyms that I neither recognized nor found interesting. I was sure that they dismissed the value of things [except in an historical context] that we fought for, that we lived for.

Because I was not a stranger to this condition of emotional dishealth , where I have the "baby" virus which temporarily leaves me feeling sorry for myself, I knew that the fever would break eventually. Pride would back it down. It always had. But still, in the wait I had this picture of me: a shuffling old man in the middle of the wrong dusty street, the earth trembling underfoot. It is festival time in Pamplona. It is the running of the bulls.

There may be no better antidote for a spell of self doubt than for someone to ask for your opinion. Thanks to this volume I am scrambling out of the doldrums as I search for the best way to express my feelings about leadership.

What makes a leader? What are the components of leadership? Can you teach it? Learn it? If you have dedicated independents, do you really need one?

I have decided to take an oblique angle on the topic and not wrestle with the questions directly. I would like instead to describe individual expressions of leadership and discreet experiences that have taught priceless lessons in courage, compassion, insight and humility. While each of these is an isolated experience, they have collectively mortised with one another over my life, paving an unmistakable path that has lead me as surely as any charismatic officer on a charger ever lead anyone.

ADVICE TO MY BROTHER

If my young brother were to tell me that he was leaving his auto parts business and was about to take a job in developmental disabilities, and was in need of advice on how to approach his new vocation in some distant corner of the world, it is easy for me to imagine how I would advise. I would not talk about the specifics of managed care. I would not touch the details of capitation, waivers, HMO's or any form of accreditation. At this inaugural conversation, tax credits would be untouched along with local government control and dealing with labor organizations. At some later date we could correspond about these and self determination, "homes of their own," circles of friends, and enemies that align themselves in other shapes.

What I would spend my time doing on the trip to the airport would be telling him stories, moving stories. I would describe chilling and evocative experiences that I have had in this field. I would share quotations and axioms that have given me strength, clarity and sense of possibility.

My ambition for my brother who had lately decided to come to this campaign would not be to send him off as knowledgeable as he could be about the technical, abstract, or even most progressive concepts of the day as much as it would be to try and launch him into an orbit of motivation and belief. I would want him to be impatient for his plane to land so he could charge his first windmill. I would want him to dream not about being the next director of his agency as much as being a crusader with an obsession, with a compulsion to change history.

TIME AND DOUBLE STANDARDS

In North America we are impatient people. This is true in growing waves in other places in the world as well but it would appear that we have become more consumed with squeezing the most out of time than the rest. We hate having our gratification put off for any length. Credit cards replaced layaway so we could enjoy now and pay later, exactly the opposite of the way our grandparents lived. Our work calendars are divided into absurdly tight segments of the business day for maximum efficiency. Parents spend inestimable time driving their children inestimable miles so that the young ones can participate in the maximum number of activities in their preciously short childhood. Waiting in lines exasperates us. Traffic jams enrage. Quietly accepting anything which prevents us from having what we want almost immediately goes against our collective nature.

I live my life existentially and like most of my friends and family, I tend to embrace more than I can hold. Whether this is good or bad is up to others to judge, what is unequivocal, however, is that when it comes to the preciousness of time and gratification where people with disabilities are concerned, we who have no great disabilities at the moment and work in this field live rather hypocritically. When it comes to people who have disabilities and their time being wasted, their opportunities being denied, and their goals being put off indefinitely, we are far more patient than we would be if we were the ones being robbed. This supreme contradiction in how we value the moment for ourselves and those who depend on us is hard to defend.

Consider these examples:

A few years ago a conference was held in a Southern state. The theme of the affair was specialized foster care for children with disabilities. The evening before the event began there was a party for presenters at the home of the local superintendent. He was an exceptionally generous and pleasant host who had laid out a marvelous spread of wonderful foods and drink. There were the finest local meats, fruits and vegetables. There were cheeses and exotic delicacies from around the world. As much imported beer and wine as one could drink. Louis the *XIV* would have felt at home.

At one point the superintendent was asked how many children he had hopes of moving from his institution [which housed over 700 adults and children] and over what period? He answered ... "I guess I would like to move about 35 over the next three years. Down here we take our time."

As we dined like aristocrats, dozens of children would be denied a nurturing family life because they would come of age before it would be their turn to move. Down here we took *their* time.

*****

A social worker in Melbourne, Australia told me once about how heartbroken she was after telling a long time resident of an institution that she would be moving to a small home in the local community. "I asked her what the first thing was that she wanted to do when she got out, and she became all excited and said, 'Oh, I want to go to the Tivoli.'" My friend said, "It just crushed me because the Tivoli was torn down 20 years ago. It was like her whole youth had passed her by and she didn't even know it."

*****

Once while working on a 10-year plan to move people out of institutions I was becoming restless with the time frame and told the project leader of my discomfort. I was about to say that I thought we should shorten the period within which we were hoping to move 1,500 people out of the institutional system that housed over 3,500. I was going to suggest that we build a plan around a 5-year period rather than 10 when he said, "Am I glad that you said something because I have been really bothered by our ambition. I think we should go for a 20-year plan. You know the old adage ... 'Slow and steady wins the race.'"

Sometime later I hunted down a book of Aesop's Fables and reread "The Tortoise and the Hare". Steady won the race. Slow had nothing to do with it.

*****

In the late 1960s I helped to move a young man, who was about my age, out of an institution into a very large group home and find him a place in a sheltered workshop. Well over 25 years went by and I found myself on a tour that stopped in at the workshop where George had entered so long ago. I frankly had all but forgotten him until I saw a lined and graying man who looked familiar. He was sitting at a bench. We greeted one another with affection and guilt.

During the time that George had entered that workshop and had been suspended in a non-career, I had traveled the world, and had received a hundred adventurous opportunities that had enriched my life. During that time while George sat system-tethered to his metal stool, six U.S. Presidents had come and gone. The country's armed forces had engaged in seven military actions on foreign soil. The Berlin Wall had come down, Germany had reunited. The Soviet Union became a memory with their hockey players hoisting the Stanley Cup.

In the years that filled the gap in our acquaintanceship, Nolan Ryan pitched seven no-hitters and retired. George Foreman won the Olympics, retired and came back to his sport as a senior citizen. When I found a better place for George I was a young man, eager, energetic. I could stay out all night and go to work the next day and not be tired. I took an early retirement two years after the meeting with George. I wanted the medical benefits assured. Because no one was bothered enough by George's youth ebbing away he went from late adolescence to middle age without ever knowing the treasure of time in between.

*****

A young woman who lived with staff support in her own apartment, was telling a visitor why it was that she preferred the current arrangement over the institutions she had lived in. "It's not just that I get what I want. It's that I get what I want when I want it."

*****

I would desperately want my brother to be struck with the immutable truth that the person with the disability is treated the same way by the clock as everyone else. The calendar pages flip at the same cadence for us all and yet we, who work in the field routinely tolerate the waste of their time, the waste of their lives and impose a patience on them that we would never accept for ourselves.

FROM ADVOCATE TO CHAMPION

I heard John McGee once say that "It's when the student is most difficult that we have to be the best teachers." I have always loved this simple truth. The prodding message is like a grandmother's maxim which seems to apply to most things in life. It especially reminds me that anyone can be an advocate when the issues are fairly easy to deal with. When the tension is light, the stakes modest, when the world is supportive, advocacy is like selling ice cream. When the times are threatening and the opponents are fierce, the fall-out the greatest, the mettle of advocacy is tested. When personal comfort and conventional wisdom suggest that one should back off, be modest in desires for people with disabilities and cautious in how we proceed, is when we have to be the best advocates.

Over the years of watching people who are the best I have noticed certain qualities in common. The best stay close to the ideals which led them to the field to begin with. They have an enormous appetite for chasing what they think should be entitled to the people they represent. They stay true to their word and they are courageous.

The best advocates raise the stakes. They have higher expectations for themselves than advocacy. They assume ownership for solving problems. They are champions.

I offer here lessons in championship.

Alex had lived in the same Michigan institution for 36 years and had no desire to leave. He was satisfied with his orderly life and his family said that he particularly found his job in the laundry satisfying. Alex had a sister who was active in the local ARC and, after hearing a speech one evening where the advantages of living in the larger community were extolled, she called a family meeting. In time Alex was consulted. He was adamant. He was not going.

Alex was a gentle man. He did not like change. He was reluctant to try anything new. He was strong willed but physically frail. Alex was petrified of heights.

After several meetings, Alex's sisters convinced him to consider a move to a home in the community. It took great persuasion and, he eventually relented to give it a trial. Once in his new home Alex unfolded like a blossom caught in a time lapse photographer's lense. He became more outgoing, more confident. He liked his new job less than the old but unlike the old Alex he told people about his feelings. He made new friends and told everyone he was much happier now, at age 70 than he ever had been. He still was petrified of heights.

In 1983 Michigan was still in the throes of controversy over moving people from institutions to single family neighborhoods. A rally was planned for the State Capitol to galvanize support among those fighting to change the old ways.

Alex was asked to deliver a speech to the throng. He had grown dramatically in the time since his big move yet he was still self conscious. He still had his fears. Again he was persuaded to do something he didn't really want to do. But, he agreed he said, because he wanted to "help somebody else out." He wrote a short speech and prepared to address the crowd on the Capitol lawn.

When Alex arrived at the State Capitol building there were over 3,000 people waiting. A high school band was playing patriotic songs. Placards with reminders about citizenship were everywhere. Alex was nervous to being with, the pulsating atmosphere made his heart pound. But the worst was yet to come. As he was lead toward the podium he could see the stairs, the 25 steep and petrifying stairs between himself and his word.

On this cool spring day an elderly gentleman, whom no one could have blamed for changing his mind, took the hands of two friends and conquered the height one trembling step at a time.

Alex's speech was succinct. It was clear and moving. In the end he asked the Governor to help people leave institutions and "let the sunshine in their lives." A prominent leader in the legislature said it was the best speech given during his career in Lansing.

*****

I was moved by a conversation I overheard on the Dybwad porch one afternoon a few summers ago. Barbara Cutler, who among her many fine credits is also the wise and lucky mother of a son with autism, was in a bit of an argument. She was in a heated exchange with a very respected professional who, at least on this point, was urging her to be realistic about what she was wanting from the system.

"For God's sake, Barbara, we can't save the whole world!" he said.

"Well, what are we here for then?" came her wonderful reply.

*****

Just after returning from an appointment with the eye doctor a friend told me about seeing a young woman in his ophthalmologist's office. The woman had two young men with her whom my friend recognized as being from one of the group homes that he was familiar with. The men were tall, well built and very energetic. They did not speak but had great curiosity which they expressed by frequently getting out of their chairs and roaming about the room. Each time the staff person would gently and calmly return them to their seats. She read to them, explained pictures to them and sang softly to them. Valiantly she tried to divert their attention from the others waiting. But periodically the men would get up and go over to someone and touch them or get too close to their faces. The young woman would always tenderly bring them back all the while offering an apology for the slight intrusion.

My friend said that no one, including himself, showed the men or the wonderful staff person any support, understanding or even common courtesy. He said, "That young girl was a marvel. We were all uptight snobs."

*****

I toured an institution with a Federal Court judge some years ago because of his wanting to experience the controversial setting firsthand. The institution was at the heart of a lawsuit that was typical of the deinstitutionalization litigation over the last 25 years. Each of the two sides had made their passionate arguments to the judge. He even appointed his own expert to make an assessment of the institution and then advise him on its place in the system of services. The whole matter had become a very explosive and emotional topic in the state and especially in the community where the institution was located. The support for maintaining the institution was overwhelming in the news media, legislature and the public opinion. The judge was under enormous pressure to side with the popular position. After all the lobbying was completed, the judge decided that he needed to take a walk.

I had been through the wards before, yet on the day of the grand tour everything was at its very best. The floors gleamed, the staff smiled, people and bustle were everywhere. The entourage was treated to a very pleasant lunch and the various programs were described by those in charge. Parents who defended the place entreated the judge to keep the institution alive. In addition to the attorneys for the state, the judges' own expert, who was a long time and trusted friend, also maintained that there was a clear and important purpose for the institution to fill.

In the end the judge graciously thanked everyone for their advice and consultation. He had become convinced that the place must close because of the persuasiveness of the argument for closure but more because as a result of the tour his heart had told him so.

*****

It was the Friday before Christmas in 1971. The Motown sound seemed to own my car radio as I shuttled residents of the Plymouth State Home and Training School back and forth across the city of Detroit. I was taking people home for the holidays and I had already made 3 trips which took about 3 hours each for the round trip. It had snowed throughout the day and the driving although not really dangerous whitened the knuckles, nevertheless.

I had taken 10 people home. They had suitcases, packages, their best clothes and the brightest smiles on board. Each trip was happy but they became increasingly tiring as the traffic thickened. Each time we made a stop, the reunion was so sweet it tugged at my heart. After a time, the combination of driving and emotion had left me drained.

I was returning from the east side after the last trip, it was snowing again. It was cold. I had worked more than a full day. The wind blew and it was grey. Melancholy was in the air. I knew that I had promised Robert that I would take him to his grandmother's house this day. But I also knew that I was tired and I could take him on Saturday, first thing. He would understand.

I began to think of the excuses which I could lean on for not following through on my promise. It was already 10:00 p.m. I wouldn't get home until after 1:00 a.m. His grandmother was probably already in bed. Robert himself was likely in bed. No one could really blame me for putting it off for a few hours. I never guaranteed that I would take Robert to his grandmother's house today. It was more or less a loose understanding.

When I pulled into the main drive of the institution I had started to feel comfortable with my plan of going home after dropping the state car off and returning the next morning for Robert. When I took the car keys to the night operator she told me that the ward charge, Mrs. Matthews, in Binet Hall, had asked that I call her no matter the time. A shiver of guilt shook my body. I worked up my nerve and called. The conversation was simple enough. It was straight from and to the heart. Mrs. Matthews was well over 60 and she told the social worker who was a third her age about life and obligation in three short sentences.

"You know you have a young man over here who has been waiting for you all evening. He said that you are going to take him to his grandmother's house. He's counting on you."

"I know." I said. "It's just taken me longer than I thought to get back because of the snow. I'm on my way."

On the short drive to the Hall from the Administration Building I was singed with shame. I felt self conscious, even cheesy. I pulled up in front of Binet and ran in through the snow. Robert was sitting on one of those hard benches in the lobby. He had his old suitcase next to him. He was dressed in the best he owned and wore a colorful headband which was popular at the time. When I saw him I acted like no selfish motive had ever crossed my mind. I asked ...

"Did you think I had forgotten you Robert?"

"No. I knew you wouldn't forget me Pro. I knew you wouldn't."

No Man is Free Until All Men Are Free

Early in 1978 a light plane crashed in the mountains of upstate New York. The plane had two people on board, the pilot and one passenger. Both were killed. People from a small town in the Adirondacks closest to the crash witnessed the explosion and knew from that moment that no one survived.

The plane had come from Florida and the single passenger on board was a young man from Grosse Ile, Michigan. Because there was a local connection Michigan news media covered the events which unfolded.

The sister of the young man from Michigan immediately made her way to the town at the foot of the dreadful mountain. She was desperate to be there when the bodies were brought down. But there was a delay because a fierce snow storm, raging for days, had became so blinding that the search up the mountains was temporarily called off. When visibility returned it would all begin again. Conditions improved slightly, then they worsened again. This pattern repeated itself maddeningly for days.

A Detroit television reporter followed the frustrated sister one afternoon as she trudged through the town valiantly and tearfully trying to get men to form a rescue party that would defy the blizzard and bring the body of her brother down off the mountain.

The image of this young woman going into the comfortable taverns of the town and standing before people who were warming themselves by their fireplaces at home, pleading with them to take on this mission, was searing. The case she made was virtually an impossible sell. Risk your life by braving wickedly dangerous conditions on a freezing mountain side to bring back the dead to an emotional sister.

In the end, however, she managed to coax a half dozen men from their comfort and safety to take on the heroic challenge. The trailing television reporter interviewed one of the men as he was packing his gear. "Why would you take on this extremely dangerous favor for people you don't even know?" he asked.

"A man lost in the mountains deserves not to be abandoned," was the simple answer.

*****

There are somewhere in the neighborhood of 50,000 people with developmental disabilities living in state run institutions in the United States alone. While this figure was once more than 4 times as many, it means little if you are one of the 50,000. In addition to this group, there are at least as many people with developmental disabilities living in private institutions and nursing homes in this country. The number in our jails is uncertain but by all popular accounts there is a disturbing non declared shame with respect to the dramatically increasing number of people with serious disabilities finding themselves in the correctional system in the United States.

In some respects the group that has been most trapped is the one which lead the way out of the institutional system to begin with. Throughout the United States there is some version of the traditional boarding home which houses untold thousands of people who were the first to leave institutions for "the mentally retarded" thirty and more years ago. Because they were high functioning they easily fit into congregate facilities that offered little supervision. Because they were capable they were never seen as requiring significant levels of funding, supports or even advocacy. The beautifully progressive concepts of the day like self determination, circle of friends, "home of your own", have largely never been visited on these pioneers. These people blazed the trail yet they have few if any of the advantages which others have who came after them. Some might suggest that where these people live and what they do is their choice. I beg to differ. It is not choice which keeps them experiencing life in a way which resembles our own in only the most primitive caricature. They live this way by default. These individuals have simply been abandoned by the professional and advocacy communities. It is as if the gulags have all been destroyed, the institutional battle over, and all that matters is to work on the refinements of inclusion, voice, and directing one's own life.

The fact is that unless we, who are wedded to this work, change the course of the tide a stratum of the population will be doomed to live and die in virtual isolation from the richness enjoyed by the rest of us. We cannot act as if the institutional matter is either already taken care of or will be rendered harmless with time. There are people who are still caught there. Time will not take care of the problem in their time. Freedom is not self executing. Citizenship does not occur spontaneously. The calendar does not give any of us another page if an infraction has occurred. There are pockets of people with disabilities all over our country who, for all practical purposes, have been disinherited. We have to correct the matter while there is still time.

Of course, there are gargantuan numbers of people with developmental disabilities living in institutions throughout the emerging former Soviet Block nations that are likely to wait for years just to be considered a low level priority as these countries try to catch up with the West in every other way. The longstanding developing nations throughout the rest of the world also beg for intervention and assistance, not just our sympathy. We are members of a global community of champions, and champions do not ignore people in distress.

In a television interview I heard James Baldwin, the expatriate American author, remind that "no man is free until all men are free." Unless we assume personal ownership for the responsibility of making all men free then the popular inclusion concepts of the day are reserved for the privileged and the lucky.

We must always be working the mountainside. We simply cannot abandon a generation of people. No one deserves that. We cannot turn our backs on the gift of being called to the rescue.

THE POWER OF ONE

A few years ago I had one of those rare moments while flipping through the television channels. I found something that moved me and continues to inspire. Lech Walesa was about to receive the highest award our county can bestow on a non-U.S.

citizen. One of the young Kennedy women was making the presentation. About this little electrician from the shipyard in Gdansk, Poland, this simple man whose tenacity toppled the first domino that lead to the collapse of the Soviet Union, she said:

"He stood in the path of history and it turned aside."

The human service mission that we are on is much less daunting than taking on the Soviet Empire. For this reason we have to take greater responsibility for the outcome and we have to accept a personal responsibility for creating a sense of comraderie that will compel people to succeed. We have to accept that each of us can control the culture within our world of work, and within our crusades. We can set the mood. We can set it with our voice, with our laughter, with the rolling of eyes, with brooding and complaining. We set it with our body language and our determination.

Whether we work in a place where people feel positive, energetic and productive, and enjoy work, or merely take a paycheck from a place that has a culture of pessimism, and whiny rivalries, it is in our control, not some central office.

An enormous part of our job then should be spent in shaping a productive and satisfying climate. We have to convince that the work is more exhilarating than exhausting, more exciting than exasperating, more dramatic than depressing. We have to help one another come to see that the tedium of the labor is worth the size of the prize. We are in the business of changing society's collective mind about the way it sees and treats a slice of its people. We are in the liberation business. It should not be a hard sell.

Unlike the auto parts trade, however, the competition in the liberation business is more a struggle for one's soul, for one's perseverance than market share. Consequently, one should be prepared to be dismissed from time to time by those who are jealous, and discounted by those who are the most pure. We can expect to be tempted to decaffeinate over advocacy and diminish the belief in our ability to achieve great things. We will be tempted by people who have already decided this for themselves.

In particular we should be wary of cynics. They orbit our lives forever. [I have come to see this as a universal truth.] The cynics come into view, usually when we feel the most hopeful and excited about something, and then they arch high above and beyond us in superior flight as we are left to question our own balance. The good thing is that we can be assured that they will drift off into the same endless trip, the same pointless trip that cynics have always locked themselves onto. We just have to resist the pull of their gravity because cynicism tends to starve optimism which is the great fuel of success.

*****

Harry Crews is an author whom I heard being interviewed on the radio a few years ago. He was talking about conversations he had with Karl Wallenda, one of the great circus performers of the 20th Century. At the time of the meeting Wallenda was 61 years old and still working the high wire. His trademark of course, in addition to the act being a family act, was that he navigated the wire 60 feet above the ground without a net.

Crews recalled how he asked Wallenda to explain why it was that he continued to perform this incredibly dangerous feat. The great Karl Wallenda answered:

"Being on the wire is living. Everything else is just waiting."

*****

For virtually everyone I know, the waiting between performances on the human services version of the high wire is welcomed, if not yearned for. Gunnar Dybwad is the single exception.

I have never known Gunnar not to be working on some speech, article, lecture, or law suit. He is always either in the middle of correspondence, preparing for a class or in the process of making a call to a self-advocate in Kenya. He is the only person that will happily answer his telephone at 3:00 AM and cheerfully run off to get the address of someone he wants you to write to. His devotion to every conceivable facet of developmental disabilities has not only been unwavering over all the years, it might be strengthening.

In some ways of all the prodigious contributions Gunnar has made to this field the most important is his example. The example of a lifetime of drive, of centered passion. His sustained familiarity with all the relevant issues, personalities and nuances in this business, the level and quality of his output, his inexhaustible curiosity about what is happening everywhere is awe inspiring. This is why he is the hero.

Another fascinating thing about Gunnar is that his mix of friends is so rich. They represent every level of official, bureaucrat, academic and advocate. They include authors, the young, the old, the brightest minds and the long forgotten. Anyone can surround themselves with people who mimic their ideas and style. The diversity in personalities, their positions on issues and their opinions about one another is evidence that Gunnar is not into cloning. It also shows that he never gives up on people. He is respectful of what they have done even if they need to do more or do it differently. He is always working on that superintendent who cannot fully embrace life outside the institution. He never relents in his crusade to convince a state commissioner to stand up to the political machine. He irrepressibly works to bring the international community together, one person at a time.

I have also always found it intriguing that while mammoth and petty rivalries have raged in this field, so many of the rivals thought of Gunnar as their mentor. It is because he has the profound capacity for being a great teacher, an inspiring conscience, and a welcoming harbor.

For the developmental disabilities community it's as if Gunnar Dybwad has been superego and comforter since time began. He has been our ballast for over half of this century. He is a throwback marvel in the computer age.

The last gasp of advice I would share with our new member of the crusade on his departure for a world that can enrich his life beyond belief would be this:

Ask yourself what you would like said about you in your 90th year. Would it be that since times were complex and politics so simple and the work so tangled that you took another job shortly after trying human services in 1998? Would you be satisfied with people saying that you quietly worked in the field until retirement than moved to a lovely home in Florida where you enjoy your leisure on the beach?

Or would you prefer that everyone talked about how the crucible of this work fed your heart and that you were still answering the phone in a resonating voice at 3:00 a.m.? And, that you were interrupted at that very hour as you prepared the guest room for another pilgrim who needed your friendship and your wisdom?

Shoot for the moon, my brother.

Shoot for the moon.

Appendix I
Curriculum Vitae of Gunnar Dybwad

EDUCATION

Doctorate of Law, University of Halle, Germany, 1934

2-year Certificate (MSW equivalent), New York School of Social Work, 1940

Honorary Degree, Doctor of Humane Letters, Temple University, 1977

Honorary Degree, Doctor of Public Service, University of Maryland, 1984

CAREER SUMMARY

1933–1941	Criminological studies in Italy, German, England and the USA
1942	Director of Clinical Services, Michigan State Institution for Delinquent Boys
1943–1951	Head of Child Welfare Program, Michigan State Department of Social Welfare
1951–1956	Executive Director, Child Study Association of America
1957–1964	Executive Director, National Association for Retarded Citizens
1964–1967	Co-Director (with Rosemary Dybwad), Mental Retardation Project, International Union for Child Welfare, Geneva
1967–1974	Professor of Human Development, and Director of Starr Center on Mental Retardation, Heller Graduate School, Brandeis University
1968–present	Professor Emeritus; international activities on behalf of the International League of Societies for Persons with Mental Handicap (now known as Inclusion International).

Professional Associations

Fellow, American Orthopsychiatric Association
Fellow, American Sociological Association
Fellow, American Public Health Association
Fellow, American Association on Mental Deficiency
Honorary Associate Fellow, American Academy of Pediatrics

Consultant, Advisory Committees

Consultant to President Kennedy's Special Assistant on Mental Retardation
US Public Health Service
US Office of Education
Social and Rehabilitation Service
President's Committee on Mental Retardation
Chair, Advisory Committee on Special Education, Massachusetts Advisory Council on Planning, Construction, Operation and Utilization of Facilities for the Mentally Retarded, President, International League of Societies for Persons with Mental Handicap

Honors

American Association on Mental Deficiency (1969, 1986, 19990)
International League of Societies for the Mentally Handicapped (1972)
C. Anderson Aldrich Award (1973)
President's Committee on Mental Retardation (1977)
National Association for Retarded Citizens (1978)
Massachusetts Psychological Association (1981)
International Association for the Scientific Study of Mental Deficiency (1981)
Kennedy Foundation International Awards Program (1986)
Pike Institute, Boston University School of Law
Foundation of Dignity, Philadelphia

Appendix 2

Concluding Remarks From Gunnar Dybwad's Response Upon Receiving an Honorary Degree of Doctor of Humane Letters from Temple University

February 12, 1977

... And now that I can look back to almost **50** years of work in what we call the field of human services, where do I see the lasting verities, which have increasingly fashioned my approach to serving persons with a handicap?

1. In dealing with the problem of human growth and development, one should never say "never." There is always change, the dynamics of which so far have not become clear to scientific exploration; no one can predict as an individual being is born, where the limits of that person's growth and development will be. I reject and resent the arrogance of bureaucratic and professional workers who predetermine another human being's potentials.
2. Men may continue trying to apply measurements to intellectual functioning, adaptive behavior, and emotional maturity, but the inherent dignity of any human being, no matter how severely disabled, cannot be quantitatively assessed and to do so in the name of ethics (as has been tried) is a mockery of that term.
3. In searching for solutions to human problems, I am more and more impressed with the overwhelming importance of one's personalized environment — for the child and the family; for the adult, in addition to his home, his own living space. Thus, home support looms ever larger on my list of priorities.
4. This leads me to underline one point of wisdom from Lewis Carroll's *Alice in Wonderland*. I have often said that all administrators should have this book on their desk for easy reference. You may recall that Alice asked the Queen, "Where shall I begin?", and the Queen answered her, "Begin at the

beginning." In the field of handicap we most certainly have failed badly in that respect. Early intervention is particularly essential for persons with disabilities who require long-term care.

5. After ten years of teaching doctoral students (whose knowledge and skills often awe me), I recognize that frequently we create or exacerbate problems by pompous words. The King's English — simple, direct language in our communications — must be more recognized as a valuable tool. Along with it comes my faith in what Adolph Meyer, the distinguished psychiatrist and co-founder of our mental health movement, called "the science of disciplined common sense." Along with it must also be mentioned the admonition Edger Doll, pioneer in clinical psychology and father of the Vineland Social Maturity Scale, addressed to his students in his last years: Don't *over*estimate the value of so-called objective tests, and don't *under*estimate the value of your own structured observations. In other words, I have come to look upon a lot of ongoing research with a very jaundiced eye, because I am convinced that to a considerable extent, the facts upon which the research is supposedly based are skewed by the fact finder's biases.

6. Much of my most significant learning in the field of disability I owe to parents of children with handicaps. But more and more I am convinced that we must listen to a far greater degree to the individuals with handicaps. For a long time we thought those with more severe disability could not learn; now we know we could not yet *know* how to teach. Similarly, what we call the inability of persons with severe handicaps to communicate may well be our ineptness in listening. So we must learn to listen, and while this is not easy for those whose hearing is going sour, try we must.

And now let me thank again Temple University for the great honor they have bestowed on me, and thank you all for your presence here. It is a great evening for the Dybwads.

Appendix 3
A Final Tribute to Rosemary F. Dybwad, Ph.D.

Hank Bersani, Jr.

This has been a volume in honor of Gunnar Dybwad, his life, his work, and his 90th birthday. Although the modest old professor has given us permission to compile this volume in his honor, he has been emphatic that the book not be about him. However, for so much of his life, so much of his work, so many of his 90 years, Professor Dybwad's life was intertwined with that of Rosemary Ferguson Dybwad. The contributors to this volume (editor included) were profoundly affected by the work and life of Gunnar Dybwad. But truth be told, as he has always pointed out, we were also all affected by her, including the professor himself. Rosemary guest-lectured in his courses, reviewed his manuscripts, made suggestions, made corrections, co-authored countless reports with him, and served as an endless source of fresh ideas and constructive criticism. It is only fitting that this book in his honor ends with a reflection on the inspiration of his life.

Rosemary Ferguson was born in 1910 — but to fully understand the power of her life, one needs to understand how it was that she was born in Indiana, but grew up in the Philippines and was a world traveler long before meeting Gunnar and setting out on their rich life together.

Scholarship and social conscience run deep in her family history. Rosemary's maternal great-grandfather, Steven Riggs was born in Steubenville, Ohio, in 1812. This was in an era when Ohio was referred to as the "West." Upon his graduation from the Western Theological Seminary, Mr. Riggs married Mary Ann Langly in 1837. Shortly thereafter, he accepted a missionary assignment in the Dakota Territory in Minnesota. Determined to work with the Dakotas in their own language, and respectful of their culture, he studied the Dakotas and their language with the fervor of a scholar. These efforts culminated in his seminal publication of Dakota grammar, texts, and ethnography.

This was followed in 1887 with a second volume, an autobiography of his life and that of his wife as they continued their missionary work — *Mary and I: Forty Years with the Sioux.*

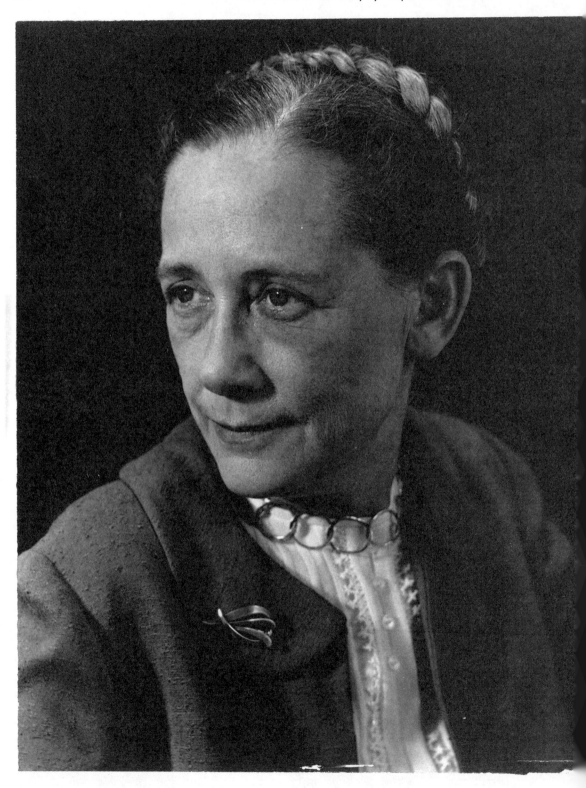

Rosemary F. Dybwad.

Rosemary's maternal grandfather, Isabella Riggs, the daughter of Steven and Mary Ann Riggs, left their home in Minnesota to travel to Ohio at the age of 16 when she entered the Western Female Seminary. This seminary later became the Western College for Women – from which Isabella, her daughter Margaret, and her granddaughter Rosemary Ferguson (Dybwad) all eventually graduated – a small, excellent institution that in more recent years was absorbed by Miami University in Oxford, Ohio.

In 1866, Isabella Riggs married the Reverend Mark Williams, and they set sail for a one hundred days' trip to China, where they spent the rest of their lives working in the missionary field. Rosemary's mother Margaret, and her twin sister Anna, were born at their parents' home in China in 1878. Margaret Williams married the Reverend John. B. Ferguson in 1907. The second of their five children, Rosemary, was born in 1910 while the missionary family was living in Indiana.

In 1925, John B. Ferguson became the pastor of the Union Church of Manila, and thus Rosemary spent her adolescent years in the Philippines, with side trips to China and Japan.

Always interested in international matters, as an undergraduate student at Western College for Women, in Oxford, Ohio, she met and became friends with several international students. They inspired her to apply to the Institute of International Education for a fellowship to attend school at a German university. She was a graduate student in Sociology at the University of Leipzig from 1931-33. While she was in Leipzig, the director of the foreign exchange program, Ingrid Dybwad, introduced Rosemary to her brother Gunnar Dybwad, who it turned out shared her interest in the English Borstal System – a new kind of reformatory for juvenile delinquents. In the next few years, she worked as a social worker in the Indianapolis Public Schools, and completed a social work internship in Indiana's Women's Prison in Indianapolis. Gunnar completed his law degree, and they returned to the U.S. They were married in January of 1934. In 1935, she returned to Germany and attended the University of Hamburg, receiving her doctorate in 1936.

During the early years of their marriage, they both worked in correctional institutions, moving to positions in several states – Indiana, New Jersey, and New York. They learned a great deal about institutions during those years. It was information that would serve them well as their careers shifted to the field of mental retardation in the next decade.

A model career woman and a dedicated parent, Rosemary terminated her employment after the birth of her son Peter in 1939, who was followed by her daughter Susan in 1941. Rosemary stayed home for years, raising children and welcoming a steady stream of international dignitaries, United Nations Fellows, and students from around the world. The Dybwad household became famous for its hospitality for decades to follow. A quick glance through the family guest book which she maintained reveals a Who's Who of famous people, not-yet-famous students, and self-advocacy leaders. The list of addresses in the book ranges from Iceland to India, from London to Sydney.

Her early professional work was in the area of women's prisons and juvenile delinquency. Beginning in 1958, she dedicated her professional career to international developments in the field of mental retardation. Today, ripples from her early efforts can be seen clearly from A to Z: from Australia to Zimbabwe, including along the way Argentina, Bangladesh, Ireland, and Austria.

When her husband became Executive Director of the National Association for Retarded Children in 1957, Rosemary turned her scholarship and energy to volunteer work. Her international experience made her a natural for looking after the increasing volume of correspondence from other nations that reached the Association's headquarters. Parents from fledgling organizations in country after country wrote NARC for advice, information, and a sense of connection. Rosemary read the letters, translated them when necessary, and offered what the NARC had to offer. From then on, Rosemary dedicated her efforts to supporting international developments in the field, and in particular, the role of voluntary organizations and Non-Governmental Organizations (NGOs). The ensuing exchange of information lead her to develop an international newsletter which contributed to the eventual establishment of the European, and later the International, League of Societies for Persons with Mental Handicaps (ILSMH). Her days with NARC clearly mark the starting point in the history of the development of an international network in the field. More than 40 years later, Tom Mutters of the International League still refers to it as "Rosemary's League." It currently lists 148 member organizations in 88 countries.

From 1964-1967, Rosemary and Gunnar were co-directors of the Mental Retardation project of the International Union for Child Welfare, based in Geneva, Switzerland. Together, they made Geneva their home. From there, they consulted in more than 30 countries around the world, helping develop programs for children with disabilities, parent organizations, and building bridges between so-called developed and developing nations. After returning to the USA, she was convinced to apply her worldwide knowledge in a new assignment — working for the President's Committee on Mental Retardation to organize an international directory of mental retardation resources.

From 1966-1978 she was active in the International League of Societies for Persons with Mental Handicap, first as a board member, and later as First Vice President.

In 1975, she was appointed to the Massachusetts Developmental Disabilities Council, and in 1976 to the Board of Visitors of Boston University's Sargent College of Allied Health Professions. She served as a consultant on International Affairs to the President's Committee on Mental Retardation, as a Visiting Scholar at the National Institute on Mental Retardation in Canada (now the G. Allan Roeher Institute), and on the Human Studies Committee of the Eunice Kennedy Shriver

Center. Rosemary was a Fellow in both the American Association on Mental Deficiency, and the American Sociological Association. The Western College Alumnae Association selected her as the winner of their 1991 service award. The Association statement said: "... she is inspired by fundamentally human concerns, and that she has always succeeded in integrating a truly international vision of human potential with a day-to-day interest in the lives of ordinary people, above all, people with mental handicaps whose own opinions on their situation are rarely consulted. She was among the earliest to insist that [they] are people first, human beings with needs, feelings and rights, fellow citizens rather than objects of charity or compassion."

Together with Gunnar, she has received numerous distinguished awards from the pantheon of disability organizations:

- The American Association on Mental Deficiency (1969),
- The International League of Societies for the Mentally Handicapped (1972),
- The President's Committee on Mental Retardation (1977),
- The National Association for Retarded Citizens (1978)
- The International Association for the Scientific Study of Mental Deficiency (1982),
- The Pike Institute, Boston University School of Law,
- The Foundation for Dignity, Philadelphia, and
- The Kennedy Foundation International Awards Program (1986).

On November 3, 1992, Rosemary passed away at home, surrounded by family and flowers from her garden, according to her wishes. She was in a room on the first floor of their home (made wheelchair-accessible years earlier, in anticipation of their frail years). The family held a small, private service at the home. Later, a large, public, special celebration of her life was held on November 24, 1992, at Brandeis University. Upon learning of her death, Victor Waldstrom, President of the League, said, "This is a sad moment in the history of our great movement."

Even in her final years, Rosemary could sit and discuss the history of the field in a way that few others can — from firsthand experience. I heard her speak of the very early days of the parent movement in the U.S., the beginnings of the International League, now called Inclusion International. She told of the power 40 years ago of parents, saying of their sons and daughters, "We speak for them." Then she would recall her trip to Sweden in 1967, and the early inspiration of self-advocacy. She would reflect on the increasing insistence by self-advocates that they be involved in international organizations beginning with being present at events, then making presentations, then serving on planning committees.

Countless followers have asked Rosemary for her advice, for what we need next. She was fond of offering two types of advice. For professionals, students, and other interested people who did not have disabilities, she would say — "Listen." She told us we need to listen better to the people we hope to serve. For self-advocates who asked her counsel, her advice was the corollary: "Speak for yourself," she would say to individual self-advocates and self-advocacy groups alike.

Dr. Rosemary Dybwad left behind a legacy that includes international travel, supporting the establishment of parent and self-advocacy organizations in dozen of nations. She produced an invaluable volume for international scholars in disability, the *International Directory of Mental Retardation Resources*, first published in 1971 and revised in 1979 and 1981. Her book *Perspectives on a Parent Movement: The Revolt of Parents of Children with Intellectual Limitations* was published in 1990 by Brookline Books, Cambridge, MA.

Although she was well known as a scholar, an international traveler, and an ambassador for the field of mental retardation, everyone who had contact with her was also taken by her warmth. Law Professor Stan Herr has called her the Gentle Giant. Friends and admirers from Bob Perske to Fred Krause, from Water Eigner to Lotte Moise and Barbara Goode each have their own favorite Rosemary story. Serving tea during frantic negotiations, marching at a demonstration for accessible bussing, nurturing weary travelers at all hours, we all remember a moment when Rosemary touched us personally.

Rosemary finished her career as a Senior Research Associate at the Heller School of Brandeis University, with a resource file that continues to be of great value to disability researchers with an eye toward international matters. Her work continues today in many forms. The Rosemary F. Dybwad International Trust provides scholarships for international travel – one of Rosemary's great passions. During her life the trust supported such seminal work as Bob Perske's trip to Sweden which resulted in the concept of "Dignity of Risk." More recently, the foundation has supported fellows' participation at numerous international conferences. The Rosemary F. Dybwad Fund supports self-advocacy and special projects, and admittedly has a preference for supporting the work of female self-advocates.

Finally, her work continues in the life of her husband, co-worker and best friend, Gunnar Dybwad. Gunnar continues to work, write, and speak for and with people with disabilities. He continues to collect and share resources. Now that she is gone, he tends Rosemary's garden.

About the Editor

Dr. Hank Bersani is on the faculty of Oregon Health Sciences University, where he holds appointments in the Department of Public Health and Preventive Medicine and in the Department of Pediatrics. He is the Training Coordinator for Special Education and Rehabilitation Counseling for the Oregon Institute on Disability and Development, and a member of the Assistive Technology program at the Child Development and Rehabilitation Center.

Dr. Bersani holds a masters degree and a doctorate in Special Education with an emphasis in mental retardation and developmental disabilities, and has 25 years of experience in service, research and training settings. Nationally, he has served as a consultant on disability issues to the U.S. Department of Justice, the President's Committee on Mental Retardation, the Presidents Committee on Employment of People with Disabilities. And spent a fellowship year working with the U.S. Senate Finance Committee on the issue of Medicaid funded services for people with disabilities.

Dr. Bersani has been honored by receiving the Franklin Smith Distinguished National Service Award from The Arc of the United States; the Mary Switzer Distinguished Research Fellowship of the National Institute on Disability and Rehabilitation Research; and the Joseph P. Kennedy Jr. Foundation Fellowship in Public Policy and Mental Retardation. He is a Fellow in the American Association on Mental Retardation. He currently serves as an editor/reviewer for major journals in the field of disabilities, including *The Journal of Disability, Health and Religion,* and *Mental Retardation.*

Dr. Bersani was a student of Dr. Dybwad's in the 1970s at Syracuse University; years later they co-taught several courses together, and more recently co-edited *New Voices: Self-Advocacy by People with Disabilities* (Brookline Books). Today, Professor Dybwad continues to be a mentor and a guide in Dr. Bersani's professional development.